LA = linoleic Ac (om6)
ALA = α linolenic Ac (om3)

- LDL - pattern A = large, fluffy
  - pattern B = small, dense

- om3 index (RBC's) ≥ 8%

- Ancel Keys: studied sat fat intake → bt, ignored om6, om3
  ? Wt if hi sat fat correlated w. low om3 ?
  [eg: Japan had lowest sat fat + lowest CHD
    But. high om3 + low om6!]

- SAT. FAT → ↓ Lp(a)
- SAT. fat → ↑ Total chol bc converts particles to large, fluffy
- om6 → ↓ Total chol bc converts to small, dense.

- Flawed: AHA recommends 10% cal as LA (om6)
    Problems: / om6 → inflammatory
        / om6 industrial seed oils, toxic
        / om6 interfers w. pw/ usp. om3
            (compete f. sa ez)

P.53 OXLAMs = oxidized linoleic Acid metabolites

?.54: Estimated Trans fat intake = 5.b grams/day.

Insight: Why ds Dean Ornish "low fat" work?
        → bc massively ↓om6 load → massively ↓ om6 & om3
                = massively ↓ infl

Praise for

SUPERFUEL

"Contrary to the goal of pervasive marketing efforts, dietary fat is fundamental for health, disease resistance, longevity, and yes, even weight loss. Dr. Mercola and Dr. DiNicolantonio deftly reveal how the specific fats we choose to eat may well be the most important dietary decision we make in terms of directing our health destiny."

— **David Perlmutter, M.D.**, #1 *New York Times* best-selling author of *Grain Brain* and *The Grain Brain Whole Life Plan*

"If you want to know the real 'fat facts,' please read *Superfuel* by Drs. Mercola and DiNicolantonio! They make a compelling and readable guide to navigate through the often confusing dietary advice regarding the types of fat to include in your diet as well as the ones to avoid like the plague. And spoiler alert: long-chain omega-3 fats from fish oil and other sources, and quality olive oils, are something you need more of, not less of, in your diet daily for perfect heart and brain health. Prepare to be amazed at what you don't know about why we are so sick. Read this book!"

— **Steven R. Gundry, M.D.**, *New York Times* best-selling author of *The Plant Paradox* and *The Plant Paradox Cookbook*; Medical Director, International Heart and Lung Institute, Palm Springs and Santa Barbara, California

"*Superfuel* is a fascinating discussion about how much of what we've learned about dietary fat is completely wrong. This helps upend much of the low-fat dogma that has dominated nutritional thinking for the last 40 years. This book is a must-read if you are interested in improving your health through diet."

— **Jason Fung, M.D.**, author of *The Obesity Code*

"If you would like to know the truth about which fats support health, which ones don't, and what foods they're found in, open this book. It's packed full of vital information for lifelong health."

— **Dr. Frank Lipman**, *New York Times* best-selling author of *How to Be Well*

"Dr. DiNicolantonio and Dr. Mercola have an incredible wealth of information and insight to explain everything you need to know about the fats that fuel your body. You'll learn which foods you should eat, which you should avoid, and how you should cook and consume your food for optimal health . . . physically, mentally and emotionally. *Superfuel* will help and heal so many people."

— **Drew Manning**, *New York Times* best-selling co-author of *Fit2Fat2Fit*

"In *Superfuel*, Drs. DiNicolantonio and Mercola offer a view of dietary fat that's powerfully perspective-shifting. They have done a deep dive into the best research available and come up with practical, accessible guidance for taking control of your health, starting right now."

— **Dr. Aseem Malhotra**, author of *The Pioppi Diet*

SUPER FUEL

ALSO BY DR. JAMES DINICOLANTONIO

The Salt Fix

ALSO BY DR. JOSEPH MERCOLA

*Fat for Fuel**

The Fat for Fuel Ketogenic Cookbook (with Pete Evans)*

Effortless Healing

The No-Grain Diet

Sweet Deception

Dark Deception

The Great Bird Flu Hoax

Freedom at Your Fingertips

Generation XL

Healthy Recipes for Your Nutritional Type

*Available from Hay House. Please visit:

Hay House USA: www.hayhouse.com®
Hay House Australia: www.hayhouse.com.au
Hay House UK: www.hayhouse.co.uk
Hay House India: www.hayhouse.co.in

SUPER FUEL

Ketogenic Keys to Unlock the Secrets of Good Fats, Bad Fats, and Great Health

DR. JAMES DINICOLANTONIO
AND DR. JOSEPH MERCOLA

HAY HOUSE, INC.
Carlsbad, California • New York City
London • Sydney • New Delhi

Library of Congress Cataloging in Publication Program

Names: DiNicolantonio, James, author. | Mercola, Joseph, author.
Title: Superfuel : ketogenic keys to unlock the secrets of good fats, bad
    fats, and great health / Dr. James DiNicolantonio and Dr. Joseph Mercola.
Description: First edition. | Carlsbad, California : Hay House Inc., 2018.
Identifiers: LCCN 2018034051 | ISBN 9781401956356 (hardback)
Subjects: LCSH: Ketogenic diet--Popular works. | Alternative therapies. |
    Self-care, Health--Popular works. | BISAC: HEALTH & FITNESS / Alternative
    Therapies. | MEDICAL / Endocrinology & Metabolism.
Classification: LCC RC374.K46 D56 2018 | DDC 615.8/54--dc23 LC record available
at https://lccn.loc.gov/2018034051

Hardcover ISBN: 978-1-4019-5635-6
Ebook ISBN: 978-1-4019-5636-3
Audiobook ISBN: 978-1-4019-5637-0

10 9 8 7 6 5 4 3 2 1
1st edition, November 2018

Printed in the United States of America

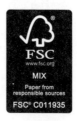

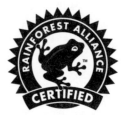

To my wife, Megan, and my two beautiful children, Alexander and Emmalyn. Thank you for always being there to support and love me.

— James DiNicolantonio

To my mom and dad—it was so hard to lose you both this past year. Thank you for your love and support throughout my life, and for creating the firm foundation in me that inspires me to educate others.

— Joseph Mercola

CONTENTS

PREFACE

A Note from Dr. DiNicolantonio

My last book, *The Salt Fix*, tackled the 40-year lie that salt is a dietary demon. If you read *The Salt Fix*, you know that contrary to popular belief, salt is not out to give you hypertension and wreck your health. It is actually an essential nutrient, and your body cannot function optimally without it.

Another popular but incorrect belief is that polyunsaturated vegetable oils (such as corn, soybean, and safflower oils) are health-promoting and that you should consume them instead of saturated fats, especially the ones that come from animals, such as butter, lard, and tallow. *Superfuel* will set the record straight.

In these pages, we will share with you evidence from human evolution showing that the human body is suited to thrive on much less omega-6 fat and much more omega-3 than most people consume today, and how this imbalance in the modern diet is the root cause of many of the chronic illnesses plaguing millions of people. We'll also show you how the fats you eat control how much fat you *store*, and which fats are the best for heart health, brain health, and fat loss.

After introducing you to omega-6 and omega-3 fats and the consequences to your health when these are out of balance, we'll walk you through how to restore optimal levels of these by choosing certain foods and supplementing wisely. Let *Superfuel* be your guide for taking back your health with a simple change in the fats you eat—no deprivation required!

A Note from Dr. Mercola

My last book, *Fat for Fuel*, presented a novel strategy for the popular ketogenic and Paleo diets. The book was aimed at helping you understand the importance of mitochondria to your overall health and how using cyclical ketogenesis could help you achieve metabolic flexibility in order to burn fat as your primary fuel. In the *Fat for Fuel* paradigm, fat is your largest macronutrient contribution—anywhere from 50 to 85 percent of your diet, depending on where you are in your metabolic cycle.

Space limitations did not allow me to go into great detail in that book as to why the *selection* of your fats is so crucial. The intention of *this* book is to fill that gap and to provide you with the solid science you need so that you can see clearly through the murky waters that many well-intentioned but confused public health authorities, physicians, and journalists have churned up over the past two generations.

INTRODUCTION: FAT CONFUSION

For decades, saturated fat was demonized. It was blamed for high cholesterol levels and clogged arteries, while medical and nutrition organizations anointed vegetable oils with a "health halo." This was because saturated fats raise cholesterol levels whereas vegetable oils (which consist mostly of polyunsaturated fats) lower them. And yet, headline after headline has come out recently claiming that you were misled: not only is saturated fat "okay" for you to eat, but it's actually *good* for you. But some of the professional nutrition organizations and government dietary agencies sharing this news are the very same ones that initially told us to stay away from saturated fats! It seems like every week the "experts" tell us something different, so what are we supposed to believe?

If you follow the 2015 Dietary Guidelines for Americans (DGA), then you would be consuming ample amounts of vegetable oils, such as cottonseed, soybean, corn, safflower, and sunflower oils, in order to lower your cholesterol levels and reduce your risk of heart disease. And in order to keep your saturated fat intake to less than 10 percent of your total calories (as recommended in the 2015 DGA), you should go easy on red meat and pork and eat fat-free or low-fat dairy products. And there's more: while the DGA emphasize consuming vegetable oils, an extremely import-ant type of fat—omega-3—is overlooked entirely. Omega-3 fat has long been considered "heart-healthy," but now not only is it not included in the DGA, it is being attacked.

In case you've missed some of the recent headlines pertaining to omega-3 fats and their role in cardiovascular health:

Reason: Rx continues w. Hi om6 intake, addp. 1-2g om3 — IN NO WAY suk-Y. achieve beneficial om3:om6,

- "Omega-3 Supplements Don't Lower Heart Disease Risk After All" (*TIME*, 9/12, 2012)

So infl continues –

- "Daily Fish Oil Supplement May Not Help Your Heart" (WebMD, 3/17/2014)

Study HAS TO include ↓↑om6 in conjunction w↑om3, monitor↑ effect w. RBC om3 index.

- "Fish Oil Claims Not Supported by Research" (*The New York Times*, 3/30/2015)

This is enough to give you whiplash. Many cardiologists no longer consider omega-3s heart-healthy, and even Dr. Eric Topol, editor-in-chief of *Medscape*, a respected clearinghouse for medical news, said, "I have an awful lot of patients that come to me on fish oil, and I implore them to stop taking it." The *Medscape* article continued, "He [Dr. Topol] called fish oil a 'no-go.' . . . 'Fish oil does nothing,' continued Topol. 'We can't continue to argue that we didn't give the right dose or the right preparation. It is a nada effect.'"

Considering that people spend their hard-earned money on fish oil supplements precisely because they're supposed to be beneficial, it would be bad enough if, as Dr. Topol said, fish oil "does nothing." But things are actually worse than that. Authorities would have us believe that fish oil isn't just neutral for health; it's actually detrimental, and has been accused of increasing risk for prostate cancer:

- "Too Much Fish Oil Might Boost Prostate Cancer Risk" (WebMD, 7/10/2013)

- "Omega-3 Fatty Acids Linked to Increase in Prostate Cancer Risk" (American Cancer Society, 7/17/2013)

So which is it: Are the omega-3 fats found in fish or krill oil helpful or harmful? Are saturated fats bad for you or not? And why do we even have to ask these questions? Why does this controversy exist, and how did we get here? And perhaps even more important: What should we do about it?

Before we begin to find answers, we need a quick detour into what exactly fats are, what they do, and which foods contain which kinds of fat.

A PRIMER ON FATS

Nutritionists and dietitians throw around terms like "saturated fat" and "polyunsaturated fat" while taking for granted that everyone understands what these things actually are. If you're not quite sure, don't worry—you're not alone. *Most* people aren't clear on which fats are which, including many journalists, and for the sake of public health, it's too bad their lack of knowledge doesn't stop them from writing articles giving you dietary advice. Unfortunately, many physicians aren't well versed in dietary fats either, and the demands on their time leave them almost no extra to keep up with the latest scientific studies and findings. As a result, too often the public—that's you—is left with little more than soundbites parroting the prevailing nutritional dogma, *even if that dogma is incorrect.*

This would be bad enough if the only thing that misguided dietary advice did was make our waistlines a little bigger. (No, it's not just your imagination, and unfortunately, your jeans didn't mysteriously shrink in the dryer). But the truth is, carrying a few extra pounds might be one of the *least* harmful things to happen to your body if you follow the advice to get most of your fat from vegetable oils. When compared to increased risk for heart disease, dementia, cancer, insulin resistance, autoimmune conditions, and premature death, being a bit heavier than you'd like is a walk in the park.

In order to make sense of nutritional guidance regarding fats, let's start with what fats are. Biochemically, fats in your food have the same structure as the fat stored on your hips, belly, and backside. And even though you might not like the way a little extra

Sat. fatty Acid: [handwritten zigzag diagram]
Mono sat. fatty Acid [handwritten zigzag diagram] (cis- "same side)

fat stored on your body makes you look, fat—in your food and in your body—is absolutely essential for good health.

The Complexity and Structure of Fats

As we dive into the complexities of why and how fats influence your health, it may be worthwhile to take a closer look at how this diverse class of biomolecules are organized and classified.

The one (and in fact only) thing all fats have in common is their insolubility in water. This is precisely what you experience when handling regular vegetable oils, butter, or lard. The reason for this water aversion stems from certain structural elements that all fats share. They are largely, but with a number of variations, made of chains of carbon atoms accompanied by hydrogen. You can think of this arrangement as a zigzag pattern dotted with "hydrogen balls" at every turn.

This "micro-architecture" is important because it makes molecules with very flexible and linear stretches. When put together, such molecules "socialize" very well, as they have the ability to stretch out and rotate to align with their neighbors. However, while such properties are shared between all fats, they are indeed a very diverse group with broad biological utility. Therefore, we will restrict ourselves to treat the dominant branch in the family tree: the glycerolipids.

That name does in itself reveal the common denominator of such fats: they all have a backbone composed of glycerol. Glycerol is a fairly short stretch of three carbons, but instead of being fully "dotted" by hydrogen, each of the carbons is attached to what is called a hydroxy group. The other structural element that all glycerolipids have in common is a structure consisting of the above-mentioned stretches of carbons and hydrogens coupled at one of its ends with what is called a carboxyl group, which makes it into a fatty acid.

Now, on this platform nature expands and diversifies by involving vast variation in the structure of fatty acids and by throwing in another structural element: the bulky and water-loving phosphate group. Through this combinatory magic, nature provides two closely

Glycerolipids 1. TGs
2. Phospholipids (PoL.)

related but still very different families of fats: the triglycerides and the phospholipids. You are probably already very familiar with the triglycerides (TGs) because they represent the kind of fat that you observe in your daily food, and it is also the stuff that can accumulate in your blood and fat cells.

Phospholipids, on the other hand, are not what you usually find in a bottle in a grocery store. In phospholipids, the water-averse fatty acids are accompanied by a large water-loving part. Therefore, their total structure takes on two personalities: a head that likes water and two water-phobic tails (think of it as a toad with two tails). That property turns into magic when such molecules are mixed into an aqueous environment.

They spontaneously form thin membranes or sheets where the heads of the molecules line up side-by-side toward the water while the tails stick together in the interior between the sandwich of the aligned heads. This structure is the basis for all life, as the border and compartments of all cells are made of phospholipid bimembranes. Therefore, the class of glycerophospholipids contains two families that share a number of common features, yet serve widely different purposes in nature. The triglycerides provide dense storage of energy while the phospholipids provide the basic structure of all cell membranes. We are made by phospholipids and fed by triglycerides.

Before we return to a more practical approach to fats, we need to explore another aspect of the structure of the fatty acids. In their simplest form they have the simple linear zigzag structure introduced in the section above. However, by making changes to the carbon-carbon bonds, much more elaborate structures can be made. The flexible zigzag structure coming from attaching only one bond between the adjacent carbons can be made rigid when one or more of the carbon-carbon connections involve two bonds.

Thus, by creating longer chains and by adding in one or more such rigid double bonds, fairly complex fatty-acid structures emerge. In nature such fatty acids have important structural and regulatory functions when incorporated into cell membranes.

This is also where the word *omega* comes into play. You may know that *alpha* and *omega* are the first and last letters in the Greek alphabet. To name the different fatty-acid structures, chemists adopted a numbering scheme for exactly where the double bond is positioned. Within the convention of starting with the carboxylic acid, the omega number simply tells you at what position from the other end of the molecule (the omega position) you will find the first double bond. So omega-3 fatty acids, omega-6 fatty acids, and omega-9 fatty acids have a double bond at position three, position six, or position nine from the omega end, respectively.

A word of caution here: The omega numbering does not imply anything about the biological function of a fatty acid, whether it is healthy or not. Omega numbers are used in naming chemical structures, and the job to elucidate how these structures interact with our biology is left to clinical investigation of each and every of such structures named.

While all living organisms can make the simpler fats, only some types of organisms are able to produce quantities of some of the more complex fatty acids. Therefore, as long as you do not starve, you will always be able to make all the palmitic acid your body needs, but in order for your body to have optimal amounts of long-chain omega-3 fatty acids known as EPA and DHA, you must obtain them from food.

Try to separate yourself from the negative connotation you might automatically feel when you hear the word "fat." Fat has been demonized for so long that you might even physically cringe a little when thinking about it—and no one could blame you, what with supermarket shelves loaded with fat-free this and low-fat that, and doctors and nutritionists having long warned us that bacon and eggs for breakfast is "a heart attack on a plate."

What is too often left out of nutrition discussions is that all fats and oils—whether they come from plants or animals—are *combinations* of the three different types of fatty acids: saturated, monounsaturated, and polyunsaturated. There are no fats or oils that are completely saturated or completely unsaturated. For example, it might surprise you to know that pork fat—including bacon fat and lard, which you probably shudder at even *thinking* about eating—is actually higher in *monounsaturated* fat than saturated fat. Moreover, the predominant individual *kind* of monounsaturated fatty acid in pork fat is *oleic acid*—the very same one touted as being responsible for the health benefits of olive oil! And the most highly *saturated* fat in our diet doesn't come from animals at all, but from a plant. That's right: it's coconut oil, which is over 90 percent saturated. Even olive oil, seemingly the only fat the disparate warring nutritional camps agree on—Paleo, vegan, vegetarian, low-carb—is around 14 percent saturated!

Saturated, monounsaturated, polyunsaturated—what do these terms mean? It's important that we get some basic facts down correctly here at the beginning so you'll easily understand what comes later. And we've got to set the record straight, because saturated fat does not come with a dictionary definition meaning "clogs your arteries," and vegetable oils aren't a one-way ticket to lifelong health and happiness.

The words *saturated, monounsaturated,* and *polyunsaturated* have to do with the chemical structure of fatty acids. For the sake of simplicity, we'll just call those fatty acids *fats*. Fats are long strings of carbon atoms joined together. But these carbon atoms have extra spaces for other atoms to attach to them too, and these other atoms are hydrogen. When all the extra spaces that can be filled *are* filled, the fat is said to be saturated—that is, it's *saturated* with hydrogen atoms. It's not because it saturates your blood vessels, in case you've ever wondered about that.

When two or more of the carbon atoms in a fat double up on each other (a double bond), it crowds out room for hydrogen. Because of this, the fat is said to be *unsaturated*, because it does *not* contain the full amount of hydrogen it would if there were no double bond. When there is just one double bond in the fat molecule, it's a *monounsaturated* fat (mono meaning *one*). When there are two or more double bonds—yep, you guessed it—that's a *polyunsaturated* fat (poly meaning *many*).

The oils we eat are some combination of saturated, monounsaturated and polyunsaturated fatty acids, because different types of fat always travel together. No fat or oil is entirely saturated or entirely unsaturated. Table I gives you a glimpse at a few different fats and oils, and their proportions of saturated, monounsaturated, and polyunsaturated fatty acid content.

Table I:
Fatty Acid Composition of Select Fats and Oils

Type of fat or oil*	% Saturated	% Monounsaturated	% Polyunsaturated
Coconut oil	91	6	3
Butter	66	30	4
Lamb tallow	58	38	4
Palm oil	51	40	9
Beef Tallow	49–54	42–48	3–4
Lard	44	45	11
Duck fat	35	50	14
Chicken fat (schmaltz)	30–32	48–50	18–23
Cottonseed oil	29	19	52
Peanut oil	17	56	26
Olive oil	16	73	11
Soybean oil	15	23	62
Sesame oil	15	41	43
Corn oil	14	27	59
Sunflower oil	13	18	69
Grapeseed oil	11	16	73
Safflower oil	9	11	80
Flaxseed oil	9	17	74
High-oleic sunflower oil	9	81	9
Canola oil	7	65	28

* The fatty acid composition of animal fats will differ slightly, based on the animals' feed (for example, grass vs. grains).[1]

Now that you know what the words actually mean, what's the *significance* of a fat or oil being saturated or unsaturated? And before we even go there, what's the difference between a fat and an oil? Fats are solid at room temperature (like butter and lard), while oils are liquid (like canola and soybean oils). *How solid* a fat or oil is depends on the number of double bonds it has. The more saturated a fat is, the harder it will be at colder temperatures, which is why beef tallow and butter are completely solid in the refrigerator, but you can scoop up cold chicken fat and duck fat easily with a spoon. Highly *unsaturated* fats don't solidify even when they're cold, while fats that are mostly monounsaturated will solidify somewhat, which is why olive oil congeals a bit if left in the fridge, but fish or krill oils, which are very highly unsaturated, remain completely liquid.

Far more important than the solid versus liquid issue is the chemical stability of the different kinds of fat. In a nutshell, saturated fats are more stable than unsaturated fats. Double bonds make unsaturated fats susceptible to detrimental chemical changes upon exposure to heat, air, and light: the more double bonds a fat has, the more susceptible it is. What this means for you in the practical sense is that some fats and oils are better suited for cooking, while others are best eaten cold—or not eaten at all. For example, as you can see in Table 1, corn oil and sunflower oil are predominantly polyunsaturated, so you wouldn't want to use them for cooking. Coconut oil and animal tallows (rendered fat) are highly saturated, so they're okay to cook with.

In case you're not sure *how* a fat or oil might be exposed to heat, air, or light, let's take a quick look. Animal fats are typically harvested from animals and then heated (rendered) to liquefy them in order to strain out stray bits of meat or bone that may have gotten mixed in and to pour the fats into containers for sale. During the rendering process, the fats are exposed to heat, light, and air, but because the animal fats contain a high proportion of saturated fatty acids, they tend to stay intact better and are less damaged from heat and pressure. Even the animal fats that have a fair amount of polyunsaturated fatty acids (such as chicken and duck fat) are relatively stable because they also have an appreciable amount of saturated fat. We expose these fats to heat, light, and air when we add them to a pan to cook a meal, but again, they're mostly stable and can stand up to the heat.

On the other hand, with the exception of coconut, palm, and high-oleic varieties of oil, oils from plants are mostly *unsaturated*. This means they're not well-suited for high-heat cooking. In order to extract large amounts of oil from things like soybeans and corn kernels—which aren't all that fatty in the first place—stunning amounts of heat and pressure are applied. You might be able to render lard or tallow in your home kitchen, the way your great-grandmother may have done, but you couldn't produce a gallon of corn or soy oil without multimillion-dollar equipment and a big factory.

These oils may be heated again in order to clarify, bleach, and deodorize them before they're bottled. (See Figure I regarding the processing of vegetable oil below.) Then, they sit on store shelves in clear plastic bottles, where they're exposed to bright lights almost around the clock. These fragile oils are exposed to the damaging trio of heat, light, and air multiple times before they even get to the store, let alone when you use them in your home cooking. If you're wondering about olive oil, let us put your fears to rest: because it's mostly monounsaturated, with only a very small proportion of polyunsaturated fatty acids, it's safe for cooking. Remember, the number of double bonds determines how "fragile" and easily damaged a fatty acid is, and monounsaturated fats have just one double bond.

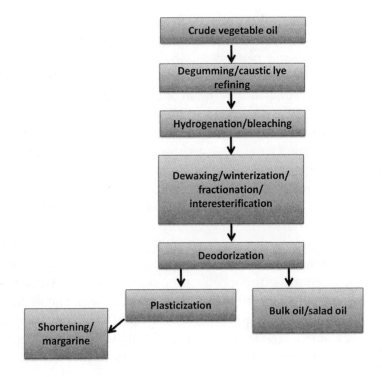

Figure I: The Processing of Vegetable Oil[2]

The precise technologies used and the order in which they are applied may differ among manufacturers, but this provides a general overview of the degree of mechanization and manipulation required in order to produce large amounts of industrial seed oils.

"Vegetable" Oils?

We call so many of these plant-sourced oils "vegetable oils," but they come from grains, beans, and seeds such as corn, soybeans, cotton and safflower seeds, and sunflower kernels. Not exactly what you think of when you hear the word *vegetable*, right? Have you ever heard of broccoli oil? Or eggplant oil?

For this reason, these oils are often called *industrial seed oils.* And in dutifully following government recommendations for a "healthy diet"—and perhaps for the specific purpose of reducing your risk for heart disease—you likely stopped buying butter and bacon and stopped cooking in old-fashioned lard and tallow, swapping out these time-honored animal fats for the supposedly healthier vegetable oils. Or if you're relatively young, there's a good chance you've never used these traditional fats at all, and have never experienced the pleasure of potatoes fried in duck fat or a piecrust made extra flaky thanks to lard.

Margarine, vegetable oil spreads, and "butter alternatives" are high in industrial seed oils, and for over a half century, doctors and nutritionists have considered these "heart healthy," particularly in comparison to animal fats. For decades, saturated fats were fingered as contributing to obesity and heart disease. In fact, it became virtually impossible to find the words *saturated fat* without the phrase "artery clogging" in front of them, as if they were all one word: *arterycloggingsaturatedfat,* right? This led to the recommendation that we should replace saturated fats with seed oils in our diets.

Industrial seed oils are high in a particular type of fatty acid called *linoleic acid* (LA). Linoleic acid is a polyunsaturated fat, the consumption of which typically results in lower cholesterol levels. Linoleic acid is considered an "essential" fat. When something is classified as "essential" in the dietary sense, it means more than simply "you need it." It means that your body can't get it by making it from something else—you *must* get it from your food. However, even though it is "essential," your current intake of LA is likely so high (primarily from the consumption of these industrial seed oils) that there's very little risk of becoming deficient in it.

Old estimates recommending that LA should make up at least 2 percent of your total calories was likely a dramatic overestimation; more recent data suggests you probably need only about one-fourth to one-half this much, or as little as 0.5 to 1 percent of total energy as LA. To put this in perspective, in the U.S., we currently consume as much as 7 to 8 percent of our total calories from linoleic acid—something basically unheard of in all of human history. In other words, there *really* isn't much danger of anyone becoming deficient.

Still, numerous dietary guidelines from health agencies around the world recommend an increased intake of linoleic acid to lower the risk of high cholesterol, intending this to reduce the global burden of heart disease. The consumption of animal fats began to decrease, and fragile, unstable linoleic acid came to dominate our diet in the form of these celebrated seed oils.

Remember, because of the industrial mechanization required to extract seed oils, these were never a significant part of the human diet until recently. They *couldn't* have been; the technology to produce them simply didn't exist. So it's a bit bizarre that nutrition advice from government agencies and, indeed, from some physicians and dietitians has been to use these oils in place of the other fats and oils that people were cooking with and eating for centuries. They didn't have any evidence at all to support this argument.

Beginning in 1961, the American Heart Association advised Americans to swap out animal fats for vegetable oils, and health agencies and government organizations around the world have continued to drive this message figuratively and almost literally down our throats. This has led to a dramatic increase in our consumption of omega-6 linoleic acid. Between 1909 and 1999, the estimated amount of linoleic acid consumed in the United States increased from approximately 2.8 percent to 7.2 percent of total calories—more than a 2.5-fold increase.[3] Seven and one-fifth of total calories from one specific type of fat might not seem like all that much, but don't be fooled: this is one of the single greatest changes that occurred in the American diet during the 20th century.

The dramatic rise in linoleic acid consumption is due primarily to the use of soybean oil. Soybean oil is high in linoleic acid, and consumption of soybean oil increased over *a thousand percent* from 1909 to 1999.[4] In the U.S. in the early 1900s, our diet contained approximately equal amounts of omega-6 and omega-3 fats. Now, however, we eat almost 30 times as much omega-6 fat as we do omega-3.[5,6]

[handwritten annotation top: "① om₃ +om₆ compete f.ez / So, it [om₆] Hi, occupies ez + ds Not allow smallrant o om₃ to be processed in pathways favorp anti-infl₂"]

The idea that a diet high in industrial seed oils is good for you is a myth. So how is it that these industrial seed oils make up such a significant portion of our total calories? Why all the conflicting information?

We believe the confusion has arisen because these two fats are involved in similar biochemical pathways inside the body, and so the degree to which omega-3 fats are good for you depends on how much omega-6 they have to compete against.

Think of it like a team of firemen trying to put out a towering inferno: even if there are plenty of firemen and multiple water hoses, if the fire is raging out of control and spreading to multiple buildings up and down the street, it will be harder for the firemen to make a dent. And the hotter the fire becomes, and the more rapidly it spreads, it gets even *more* difficult for the firemen to have an impact. It's not that the firemen aren't doing their jobs; it's just that they can't compete against the power of the out-of-control fire. Omega-3 and omega-6 fats work the same way: the more omega-6 fats in your diet, the harder it is for the beneficial effects of the omega-3s to have any impact.

[handwritten annotation left: "②Studies Not legit unless they use actual om₆ om₃ levels + document om₃ sufficiency"]

And make no mistake: the modern diet is *loaded* with omega-6. Many of the studies that concluded omega-3 fats have no impact on certain disease processes ignored the role of excessive omega-6 in the subjects' diets. It's not that omega-3s "do nothing," it's that it's almost impossible for them to make a difference against the surfeit of omega-6 they have to work against. It would be like the firemen trying to put out that enormous fire using coffee cups.

With this in mind, let's take another look at those studies that concluded that omega-3s do nothing for health. In order to offset the amount of omega-6 in most people's diets today, the studies would have had to give people about 4 grams of omega-3s. But most studies used about 1 gram *or even less*.

It shouldn't surprise anyone that the tiny amount of omega-3 wasn't enough to show any benefit in the context of so much omega-6. On the other hand, in Italy and Japan, where the omega-6-to-omega-3 ratio is around 4:1[7]—a world apart from the approximately 30:1 ratio in the U.S.[8]—you see far different results. In those studies, the health benefits from omega-3s are obvious.

TYPES OF OMEGA-3 FATS

As mentioned earlier, linoleic acid is a subtype of omega-6 fatty acid. Similarly, the category of omega-3 fats encompasses several different subtypes of fatty acids. The ones you're likely most familiar with are alpha-linolenic acid (ALA), eicosapentaenoic acid (EPA), and docosahexaenoic acid (DHA). ALA is the omega-3 found mostly in green vegetables, nuts, and seeds (such as flax and chia seeds). EPA and DHA are primarily found in fatty fish, shellfish, and krill, as well as in smaller amounts in the fat of grass-fed ruminant animals (cattle, sheep, goats, deer) and in egg yolks, especially if the hens' feed includes fishmeal or flax or chia seeds. The hens convert the ALA from these seeds into EPA and DHA. EPA and DHA molecules are longer than ALA molecules, so EPA and DHA are sometimes called "long-chain omega-3s," or "long-chain marine fats," since they come mostly from seafood. Paleolithic

Alpha-linolenic acid, like linoleic acid, is also an "essential" ALA fat that your body does not make, so you need to get it from your ~14g. diet. Evidence indicates that during Paleolithic times, our hominid ancestors consumed around ten times as much ALA as we do today (about 14 grams a day)[9,10] versus the 1.4 grams[11] we consume per day in modern times). This is the opposite of what's happened with omega-6, where we now consume far more omega-6 and far less omega-3 than we ever did before.

While ALA is an essential fatty acid, EPA and DHA technically are not, because your body can *convert* ALA into EPA and DHA. For this reason, ALA is often referred to as the "parent" omega-3. The trouble is this conversion is not all that effective in most people. Most of us are able to convert only about 5 percent of ALA to EPA and just 0.5 percent to DHA, though women of reproductive age are able to convert 21 percent of ALA to EPA and 9 percent to DHA.[12] Considering the tiny amount of ALA you typically start with in your diet, the amounts of EPA and DHA you end up with is miniscule. Your omega-3 intake is so low that EPA and DHA should be considered "semi-essential," particularly because while ALA has some beneficial effects in your body, EPA and DHA are far more potent and are required for certain biochemical jobs that ALA simply cannot perform.

If EPA and DHA are so important for our health, why do our bodies convert only such small amounts of ALA into these longer chain omega-3s? There are two main reasons: First, ALA intake during Paleolithic times was extremely high, so even with such low rates of conversion, the sheer *amount* of ALA would still have provided ample amounts of EPA and DHA. Second, our intake of EPA and DHA during Paleolithic times was also high—about 2,000–4,000 mg per day.[13,14] But now, our low intake of ALA, combined with our ineffective conversion of ALA to EPA and DHA, means that EPA and DHA should be considered "conditionally essential," since most people are likely deficient in these critically important fats. If you want to match your EPA and DHA intake to the amounts we evolved on—the amounts you likely require, and that humans were eating all along until very recently, and long before anyone ever heard of heart disease or obesity—you would need to increase your intake of ALA, EPA, and DHA *tenfold*.

Why are EPA and DHA so important? Simple: deficiencies of these fats, especially when coupled with an overabundance of adulterated omega-6 fats (mainly from industrial seed oils such as soybean, cottonseed, corn, and safflower oils), drive many of the chronic, debilitating, and degenerative diseases that now afflict the industrialized world. Recent research has linked an excessive intake of industrial seed oils (high in omega-6) with cardiovascular disease, chronic degenerative diseases, dementia, and even diabetes and obesity.

A lack of omega-3s on top of a diet high in adulterated omega-6 increases risk for autoimmune diseases including celiac disease, Crohn's disease, ulcerative colitis, and rheumatoid arthritis, asthma and other lung diseases (such as chronic obstructive pulmonary disease, or COPD), allergies, neurological disorders

Paleolithic
EPA+DHA
~4 g.

(multiple sclerosis, Huntington's disease, Parkinson's disease), and diseases of the eye such as age-related macular degeneration.

new

An increased intake of omega-6 fats from industrial seed oils may also lead to increased appetite, hijacking our sense of fullness and causing us to overeat. In individuals affected by the digestive and intestinal conditions mentioned above—celiac disease, Crohn's, and colitis—damage to the intestines that impairs the absorption of food and nutrients may result in vitamin and mineral deficiencies that further reduce the body's ability to convert ALA to EPA and DHA. With more and more people being diagnosed with these conditions, this is a significant issue.

On the other hand, having adequate omega-3 fats to balance your omega-6 fats helps keep inflammation in check, helps spur the growth of neurons in your brain to support memory and cognitive function, allows for healthy communication between your brain and your muscles, and supports healthy blood vessel function (for proper blood pressure regulation) and proper overall heart function. There's almost no body system that *doesn't* need an adequate supply of omega-3 fats, both as structural components (they're building blocks of cell membranes) and as signaling molecules. **We've got to correct the imbalance of these fats on our plates and in our bodies if we want to *thrive*, not just survive.**

As you age, you become more deficient in some of the vitamins and minerals required to convert ALA into the long-chain omega-3s. Insulin resistance—an exploding epidemic—also interferes with your body's already low capacity to convert ALA to EPA and DHA. Like a car tire losing air slowly over time, the supply of long-chain omega-3s decreases as you get older—right when you need these healthy omega-3 fats the most. In contrast, omega-6 continues to flood in, further diluting the dwindling omega-3 supply, and contributing even more to your body's burden of inflammation.

(A) ALA → EPA, DHA
conversion ↓ w/ ↑ omb
— ↑ Ins. R. ** worsens w. age
— ↑ nut. defs.
— " AGE "

So What Do We Do Now?

The truth is that in advising you to eat plenty of vegetable oils, doctors, nutritionists, and government "experts" have been recommending precisely the wrong dietary fat while remaining largely silent about the right one. Well, maybe not "wrong" and "right," since you do need both omega-6s and omega-3s, but what should be emphasized is that you need to be doing almost the opposite of what the guidelines suggest: much *less* omega-6 from vegetable oils and much *more* omega-3 from *fatty* fish, pasture-raised meats, or egg yolks. (Remember, omega-3 is a *fat*; you won't get much of it by sticking with fat-free foods.)

That's where this book comes in. *Superfuel* sets the record straight on these issues and will help you make sense of the myths and misconceptions about so-called "heart-healthy" vegetable oils. You've seen headlines and magazine covers proudly proclaiming that "butter is back," and you can stop throwing egg yolks in the garbage while you eat egg-white omelets. But is *that* true? You've been fooled before. What should you believe about fats? *What are the facts?*

Superfuel will be your guide. In the chapters that follow, you'll learn:

- Our recommended Cyclical Ketogenic Eating Pattern
- How and why government and private-sector health organizations recommended that you cut back on animal fats and consume more vegetable oils, and how this may be harmful for your health
- Why your body needs a lot more omega-3 fats than most people are getting, and why many are at risk for omega-3 deficiency
- Why many of the negative health effects that have been blamed on saturated fat may actually be due to industrially processed vegetable oils

- How much omega-6 and omega-3 fat you should be eating to keep you thriving and living well into your golden years—and which foods are good sources of them

- How certain medical conditions, medications, and other lifestyle issues influence your risk for omega-3 deficiency

- How a high omega-6/3 ratio might lead to diabetes, weight gain, and obesity (hint: it's not all about cutting back on carbs!)

- How you can measure your omega-3 levels to see if you need more in order to reduce your risk for chronic degenerative illness

- How to choose the healthiest forms of fat, including which foods to make part of your diet, which oils to cook with, and which supplements to take (if you've felt overwhelmed in the supplement aisle, you won't anymore!)

Superfuel is just that: a guide for fixing your fat balance to help you stay free of chronic illness or to help you recover if you're already living with one. Optimize your fats, maximize your health!

CHAPTER 1

HISTORICAL PERSPECTIVE: DEMONIZING THE WRONG FAT

Throughout much of human history, people valued fat in their food. Today, hundreds of thousands of calories are available 24 hours a day at the nearest grocery store, and we can use our phones to order a bounty of food to be delivered right to our doorstep. But it wasn't always like that. Until very recently, wars, natural disasters, and other unforeseen events meant that people were never far away from a famine, or at the very least, a disruption in their normal diet. For this reason, fat—which provides more calories than protein or carbohydrates—was prized as an energy source. After all, that's what calories are—measurements of the amount of energy stored in food, and they used to be considered a *good* thing.

It wasn't by happenstance that our ancestors waited until fall to slaughter the animals intended for food: they let them fatten up during summer and early autumn, so there would be plenty of delicious and energy-rich fat when they were killed. And let's not forget that as recently as the 1940s, our grandmothers judged the quality of milk delivered in those quaint glass bottles by the thickness of the rich cream layer on top. How did we go from valuing fat as something to be savored and enjoyed, something that was *necessary,* to crowding supermarket shelves with low-fat and fat-free products?

The demonization of dietary fat in general, and saturated fat in particular, started in the mid-1950s. This is when a researcher named Ancel Keys published a study that seemed to indicate a positive association between the consumption of calories from fat and death from degenerative heart disease—in other words, the higher a population's dietary fat intake, the greater their rates of death from heart disease.[1] This was a landmark known as the Six Countries Study. Keys actually used data from 22 countries, and when data from the 16 countries Keys omitted in his study was incorporated, the association between fat and heart disease became much weaker.[2] Not long after, a British researcher named John Yudkin, M.D., would show that consumption of refined sugar tracks tightly with dietary fat—that is, populations with a high fat intake often also have a high sugar intake—indicating that sugar, not fat, could have been the cause of Keys's findings.[3]

Regardless of whether Keys or Yudkin had the stronger argument, these types of studies can never prove a causal effect between saturated fat and coronary heart disease (CHD), because they are *observational* in nature.[4] In health and nutrition research, an observational epidemiological study is one in which researchers look at a population, make observations about what they eat, how they live, and their health outcomes, and then extrapolate those observations into general *hypotheses* about potential connections between the former and the latter. But until these hypotheses are proven through scientific experiments, they remain hypotheses— nothing more than educated guesses.

As an example of observational epidemiology, people living in Mediterranean regions are often cited for their excellent health and long lives. This is typically attributed to the consumption of olive oil, or a diet rich in fresh vegetables, or even to moderate amounts of wine. But it could just as easily be due to infrastructure that requires much more walking than riding in cars, to the fresh air and beautiful scenery of the Mediterranean coast, to the sense of community and respect for elders in the region, or to some completely unknown factor. Epidemiology is great for generating hypotheses, but it is not reliable for determining which factors are responsible for the observed outcomes.

After Keys' Six Countries Study was published, another researcher, Edward Ahrens, became one of the first to show that when people swapped out animal fats in their diet in favor of highly processed industrialized plant oils (especially corn, safflower, or cottonseed oil), their cholesterol levels went down.[5,6,7] Moreover, the fats that raised cholesterol levels the most were coconut oil and butterfat, which are both highly saturated fats. Ahrens's findings provided plenty of ammunition for Keys to implicate saturated fats as a cause of high cholesterol.

Not long after, in 1961, a study was published indicating that elevated cholesterol was a key risk factor for CHD.[8] This was one of the sparks that lit the fire that became known as the "diet heart hypothesis." If high cholesterol levels were a major cause of heart disease, and if saturated fats increase cholesterol levels, saturated fats must therefore cause heart disease. And since polyunsaturated fats (mostly from vegetable and seed oils) were known to *lower* cholesterol levels, it was then assumed that they were "heart healthy." **But just because A (saturated fat) leads to B (higher cholesterol levels), and B is *associated* with C (CHD), that doesn't mean A (saturated fat) *causes* C (CHD).**

Despite the clear flaws in this shaky hypothesis, in 1961 the American Heart Association (AHA) officially recommended that Americans replace their intake of animal fat with vegetable oils.[9] The diet heart hypothesis grew from a small fire to a towering inferno that blazes out of control even now, no matter how much

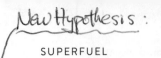

water we pour over it. To see this for yourself, peruse the butter section of your local supermarket next time you're there. The shelves are so crowded with margarine and vegetable oil spreads that it can be difficult to even *find* real butter.

So What's the Real Cause of CHD?

The real mechanism for how saturated fat increases cholesterol levels is still being debated, but it's thought to be caused by a reduction in low-density lipoprotein receptor activity in the liver. Low-density lipoprotein (LDL) is the form cholesterol takes as it moves through your blood, and if there are fewer receptors for LDL, or their activity is decreased, then the LDL particles and the cholesterol they carry accumulate in the blood instead of being taken up by the liver.[10] Polyunsaturated fats have the opposite effects on LDL receptor activity—they increase it, which lowers LDL in the blood.[11,12]

These are plausible mechanisms, but there's a problem: the increases in cholesterol levels from dietary saturated fat in animal studies occurred only when intake of omega-3 fats was low.[13] In other words, a low omega-3 intake was the more likely factor contributing to high cholesterol, and not saturated fat intake per se. At the very least, this should have led to a slight refinement of the diet heart hypothesis: **A (low omega-3 intake) leads to B (high cholesterol), which associates with C (CHD).**

But unfortunately, like so many other missed opportunities in the history of nutrition science, this didn't happen. Nuance and detail were ignored in favor of pithy sound-bites.

Early research by Keys and Hegsted that implicated saturated fat as a cause of high cholesterol (called *hypercholesterolemia*) did not take into account background omega-3 intake. Deficiency in omega-3 fats likely contributes not only to hypercholesterolemia, but also to increased inflammation, abnormal blood clotting, and CHD.

During the following decades, the diet heart hypothesis led to the demonization of milk, cheese, butter, pork, and beef, because the saturated fats in these foods could raise cholesterol levels. But not everyone believed that saturated fat was harmful. In fact, there was a "cholesterol controversy" among the scientific community that persists to this day, with many respected researchers and physicians declaring that neither saturated fat nor high cholesterol levels are harmful for the heart.[14]

Nonetheless, the first edition of the U.S. Dietary Goals, published in 1977, contained the federal government's first official recommendation that all Americans restrict their intake of saturated fat and increase intake of polyunsaturated fat up to 10 percent of total calories—recommendations that have been upheld with each five-year update of the dietary guidelines beginning in 1980.[15,16] So, since 1977, Americans have been indoctrinated with the idea that polyunsaturated fats are helpful, and strongly encouraged to avoid the demonized saturated fats.

The theory was that this would lower cholesterol levels and, as a result, reduce risk for heart disease; but as we now know, when omega-3 intake is low and omega-6 intake is high—as they typically are among the general U.S. population—lowering saturated fat intake results in increased synthesis of substances that promote inflammation and decreased synthesis of anti-inflammatory substances, which could ultimately lead to *increased* risk for heart disease—precisely the opposite of what this recommendation was intended to do!

What we've looked at so far is just the tip of the iceberg when it comes to weak nutritional science. And since official government recommendations on diet affect everything from hospital food to school lunches to what we see on store shelves and generally think of as "healthy," let's dive into a bit more of the research and see if what we *thought* we knew about fat stands the test of time, or whether, in fact, it's time for a major update.

VEGETABLE OILS AND OMEGA-6: NOT AS HEART-HEALTHY AS YOU THOUGHT

A very large, long-term diet study, called the Nurses' Health Study (NHS), found as much as a 32 percent reduction in CHD when subjects increased their intake of polyunsaturated fats. It was also estimated that replacing 5 percent of total calories from saturated fat (SFA) with polyunsaturated fats (PUFA) or carbohydrates would reduce the risk of CHD by 42 percent and 17 percent, respectively.[17,18] A 42 percent potential reduction in heart disease risk is pretty great, so when these results were published, just about everybody was pretty convinced of the notion that omega-6 fat, which you mostly get in the form of linoleic acid (LA) from vegetable and seed oils, was good for the heart.

However, these findings, once again, were observational in nature, so they are unable to prove causation. Additionally, estimates of PUFA intake were based on dietary questionnaires, which ask you to indicate how much of certain foods you consumed and how frequently you consumed them over some specific period of time. If you have a hard time remembering what you had for lunch three days ago, imagine trying to recall what you've eaten during the last 20 years, which was one of the follow-up points in the Nurses' Health Study. At best, these types of questionnaires generate extremely general ballparks of people's food consumption; at worst, they're entirely useless. Either way, they're a poor measure of what people actually eat, and they certainly cannot be considered ironclad evidence.[19]

Recommendations to replace saturated fat with omega-6 LA also came from studies showing that low LA and high SFA in the blood is associated with increased risk for metabolic syndrome, insulin resistance, and inflammation.[20] It's true that lower levels of LA in the blood are consistently associated with greater risk for CHD, death from CHD, and all-cause mortality,[21,22,23] so these findings have been used to promote the idea that LA is good for the heart and to encourage increased consumption of vegetable oils. But what wasn't readily known at the time was that inflammation oxidizes LA, creating oxidized LA metabolites, thereby lowering LA levels in the blood.[24,25] In fact, in one of the studies looking at LA in the blood, when the researchers adjusted for other relevant factors, low levels of LA were *not* strongly associated with an increased risk of death.[26] This suggests that inflammation can cause low LA levels in the blood and that the inflammation, rather than a low dietary intake of LA, drives the higher risk of CHD and death. Low levels of linoleic acid in the blood are likely a marker of increased inflammation in your body, and don't necessarily reflect the amount of this fat in your diet. So if you have a low blood level of linoleic acid, it would be better for you to reduce the inflammation, rather than consume omega-6 rich vegetable oils.

The amount of certain fats you eat doesn't automatically correlate with the amount of those fats that end up in your bloodstream. The human body just isn't that simple. After all, if you eat a lot of spinach, your blood doesn't turn green. Compounds in the foods you eat go through an array of biochemical processes that significantly alter their structure and numbers before and even after they enter our blood.

MEDITERRANEAN DIETS

The Mediterranean region has long been known for a low risk of cardiovascular disease, diabetes, cancer, and depression,[27] and the Mediterranean diet's fame goes back to that familiar figure, Ancel Keys, along with his epidemiological research from the 1950s and 1960s.[28] Keys looked at 16 areas in seven countries and found that Mediterranean areas (Italy, Crete, Croatia's South Dalmatia) had lower rates of heart disease than the U.S. and Northern Europe.[29] Japan was also noted for a very low rate of heart disease. Based on this research, which was published as the Seven Countries Study, Keys concluded that saturated fat was "the major dietary villain."[30] Left out of the study, however, was that the Mediterranean populations Keys cited didn't consume large amounts of industrial seed oils. Plus, Med. pops likely hd hier
- om₃ (seafood)
- they stuck f olive oil over seed oils

The trouble was, there wasn't just *one* Mediterranean diet pattern. Diets varied from country to country, and not all regions in which people lived long lives and had low rates of heart disease avoided meat or dairy. Think about France and Italy: they weren't exactly eating low-fat Brie or fat-free prosciutto!

While the Seven Countries Study was used to further demonize saturated fat because of its role in raising cholesterol levels, omega-3 fat intake was not even addressed; only saturated fat, monounsaturated, and total polyunsaturated fat intakes were reported in dietary analyses.[31] So the Seven Countries Study could not say for sure whether the higher rates of heart disease in the U.S. and Northern Europe were being driven by these populations consuming more saturated fat or less omega-3. Had omega-3 intake been measured, we might be blaming a low omega-3 intake, and not saturated fat, for the scourge of heart disease.

Researchers swept all this nuance under the rug, and saturated fat alone received the blame for the difference in health between Mediterranean countries and regions with higher rates of coronary heart disease. If this were a trial accusing saturated fat of crimes against heart health, any intelligent jury would've laughed this "evidence" right out of the courtroom.

OTHER RESEARCH ON DIETARY FAT

The Mediterranean diet is just one of many eating patterns that has been studied in hopes of identifying individual factors that either help or harm health in general, and cardiovascular health in particular. Unfortunately, the weaknesses that plague the research on the Mediterranean way of eating aren't unique to that region, and Ancel Keys wasn't the only scientist who jumped to false conclusions that eventually became the dietary laws of the land. Let's take a look at findings from other countries and see if they support the diet heart hypothesis or if they have more holes than a piece of Swiss cheese.

Earlier it was noted that Japan was recognized for having a low rate of heart disease. But it wasn't just low. In the late 1960s Japan was ranked *lowest* for deaths from coronary heart disease—*and* lowest for consumption of saturated fat.[32] Seems like a slam-dunk, then, right?

The lowest intake of saturated fat and the lowest rate of CHD deaths. But remember, this is only an association. Just because these two things occur together doesn't automatically mean that one causes the other. Along with their low saturated-fat intake, the Japanese also had a very low intake of omega-6 fats and a high intake of omega-3. But when Japanese people immigrated to Hawaii, their risk of CHD increased. Keys blamed this on an increase in their saturated fat intake, but it just as well could have been due to a reduction in the omega-3s the Japanese were accustomed to eating in their seafood-rich diet.[33,34] *or* †omg·fr. American diet?

A number of other epidemiological studies found associations between higher cholesterol levels and increased risk for CHD,[35] but many other studies did *not* find this association. Despite this inconsistency, the ones that did find an association were used as further ammunition supporting the idea that saturated fat was dietary enemy number one. In nutritional science, this is known as "cherry-picking." It's a dangerous practice in which researchers focus on the studies and data that support their hypotheses while downplaying or altogether ignoring the ones that don't. Research on dietary fats is rife with cherry-picking, which is one reason why there are so many conflicting headlines about diet these days.

(2009) Peter Parodi· Has↑ assoc btw SFAs, serum chol + CHD bit. overemphasized?

Cholesterol Confusion

Parodi noted↑ coc. oil → ↑LDL but even ↑↑ HDL -

Years later, when a larger number of studies had been published, researcher Peter Parodi concluded that the epidemiological studies—the ones that can only create hypotheses, and not establish cause and effect—did not support a role for saturated fat in causing heart disease. In fact, Parodi noted that while saturated fats increased LDL (the so-called "bad" cholesterol), they also increased HDL (the "good" cholesterol) even more if the saturated fat is coconut oil.

Sat fat = ↑T.C, ↑LDL, ↑HDL } HDL, Lp(a) correlate btr w.
= ↓Lp(a) } CHD risk than LDL,TC.
SUPERFUEL
= Converts small dense → large fluffy
pattern pattern

Additionally, saturated fats had another potential benefit: they decrease small, dense LDL particles and another type of lipid called *lipoprotein(a)*,[36] both of which are now believed to be better indicators of cardiovascular risk than total cholesterol or LDL. Based on a broader view of the blood lipid changes that occur with varying intakes of saturated fat, it was shown that indictors of heart health may actually *improve* with a greater saturated-fat intake, especially if that saturated fat replaces sugar and other refined carbohydrates.[37]

Remember that "saturated fat" is an umbrella term for a mixture of a group of different individual fats, each with its own unique properties. Some of their properties result from the number of carbon atoms in the fats. For example, with regard to raising total cholesterol and LDL levels, lauric acid (12 carbons), is more potent than myristic acid (14 carbons), and substantially more potent than stearic acid (16 carbons).[38] What is conveniently ignored is the intriguing fact that lauric acid also increases *HDL* the most. Most of the raising effect of lauric acid on total cholesterol comes because it typically raises HDL, which is why an increased intake of saturated fat can actually result in a decreased ratio of total cholesterol to HDL—and this ratio is a much more powerful predictor of CHD risk than LDL.[39] Talk about "an inconvenient truth."

Another inconvenient point is that the famous Framingham study—a very long-term epidemiological study of a population in Framingham, Massachusetts—showed that low intakes of saturated fat and cholesterol were associated with an increase in small-dense LDL particles, which, again, are a more powerful heart disease risk factor than LDL as a whole.[40] (You're probably accustomed to seeing "LDL" on a lab printout from your doctor, but there isn't just one kind of LDL. There are several subtypes, each with its own characteristics and effects—kind of like how there are several different types of saturated fat.)

At the same time, other studies showed that a higher saturated-fat intake is associated with an increase in large-buoyant LDL particles and a decrease in small-dense particles.[41] This is key, because a preponderance of small-dense LDL particles (referred

Handwritten annotations:

LDL — Type A - large, fluffy pattern
— Type B - small-dense pattern - ② problems
Type B ± mr. likely t. penetrate bsr, well
∵ "persist" ↓ 15 → longer time t.b. oxidized

Historical Perspective: Demonizing the Wrong Fat

to as pattern B) is believed to be more likely to be harmful for cardiovascular health than a preponderance of large-buoyant particles (pattern A). The reason for this is that small-dense LDL particles can penetrate artery walls more easily than the large-buoyant particles.

Small-dense LDL particles also remain in the bloodstream longer, which increases their susceptibility to oxidation, a type of biochemical damage.[42] You've seen oxidation, like when certain metals rust or when an apple or avocado turns brown when exposed to air. This process also happens inside the human body, and lipoproteins that carry cholesterol can become similarly damaged, as can DNA and structural fats in our cell membranes.

Researchers have found that the majority of studies show a positive association between elevated small-dense LDL particles and CHD risk—the greater the amount of small-dense LDL, the greater the risk for CHD.[43,44] And so when people cut back on saturated fat, which generally causes an increase in the harmful, small-dense LDL particles, they may actually be increasing their risk for heart disease. One study even showed that men with pattern A (large-buoyant) LDL particles who go on a low-fat, high-carb diet show an increase in those harmful pattern B (small-dense) LDL particles. As if that wasn't a big enough nail to drive into the coffin of the saturated-fat-is-bad-for-you myth, in these men, the low-fat, high-carb diet also raised triglycerides and lowered HDL,[45] indicating a higher risk for cardiovascular disease.

Like everything else we've discussed so far, this isn't a simple black-and-white issue. High triglycerides on their own may be problematic for heart health. Low HDL may be problematic for heart health. But taken together? The risk of cardiovascular disease is multiplied, not added. A low-fat, high-carb diet will *increase* your cardiovascular risk, **not lower it.**

This is especially true if saturated fat is replaced by refined carbohydrates, a swap that induces a shift from the relatively benign large-buoyant LDL particles to the more harmful small-dense ones. So if you spent a few years—decades, maybe—banishing butter or cream cheese in favor of fat-free orange marmalade or grape jam on your bagel, you were unknowingly taking part in a dietary experiment that might have compromised your heart health. So much for following those official dietary guidelines.

Clinical Trials:
Where the Research Gets Real

Most of the research we've looked at so far was observational and epidemiological in nature. Let's switch gears now to look at clinical trials. Protocols for clinical trials in nutrition research vary, but generally speaking these are studies in which two or more groups are assessed for various health issues or nutrient statuses; then they either follow their normal diet and lifestyle habits or implement some kind of change for a specified period of time. At the end of the study they are assessed again to see what differences, if any, have resulted. Sometimes studies are designed to look for specific outcomes, like whether a low-carb diet results in more weight loss than a low-fat diet or whether vitamin D supplements reduce risk for osteoporosis.

These studies typically produce more reliable findings than epidemiological surveys, but they still have their weaknesses. The biggest of these is that it's almost impossible to control for all the factors that might have an effect on health—factors completely unrelated to the diet or supplement changes, such as subjects' socioeconomic status, amount of exercise, quality and quantity of sleep, and level of education, just to name a few.

It's also difficult to control for issues that *are* related to diet. For example, if only one change is made, such as reducing intake of red meat, what about all the *other* parts of subjects' diets? They're likely not all eating and drinking the exact same things to begin with, and as we've seen, foods and nutrients don't exist in a vacuum. They interact with each other so that their effects are determined in part by what they're consumed *with* and in the context of the diet and lifestyle as a whole. Unless these things are controlled for, it's possible for study results to show connections that aren't really there.

Also - if study decreases sth → mns sth else in diet ↑, eg ↓sat. fat replaced w CHO or ↑mb make hlth worse!

Researchers understand this and try to control for it—to level the playing field, so to speak. But it's not possible to completely neutralize *every* factor that might play a role in the results. Nevertheless, with the exception of double-blind, placebo-controlled studies (which are virtually impossible to do with diets; you know whether or not you're eating more broccoli), these types of clinical trials—called interventional studies—are among the best tools we have for now. So let's look at a few of the more famous ones related to saturated and polyunsaturated fats. Were their findings cause for major changes in the American diet, or were they much ado about nothing? FMHS (1959-1971) Finish Mental Health Study

The Finnish Mental Hospital Study (FMHS) has consistently been used as evidence that industrial seed oils are good for heart health, as subjects who had an increased intake of these seed oils showed a lower risk of death from CHD. However, there were serious flaws in this study. The FMHS was a primary-prevention trial conducted in middle-aged men in two mental hospitals from 1959 to1971.[46] "Primary prevention" means preventing the *first* occurrence of something, like a heart attack or stroke. (Secondary prevention means preventing a second instance.) In one hospital, subjects were put on an omega-6-enriched diet in which butter was replaced with PUFA-enriched margarine and whole milk was replaced with milk fortified with soybean oil . . . *Yum!* Subjects in the other hospital were served the normal hospital diet, without saturated fat being swapped out for omega-6.

At the time, margarine was a major source of artificial trans fat, and it was removed in the omega-6 intervention group. So the "omega-6" intervention wasn't just a reduced omega-6 intervention but also a reduced artificial-trans-fat intervention, and this could have easily skewed the study's results in favor of omega-6. (Artificial trans fats are created when liquid oils are chemically manipulated to behave more like solid fats—this is how margarine sticks made from corn and soybean oils are solid at room temperature—and they *definitely* raise LDL levels.)

And then, the diets were switched after six years, and patients were allowed to come in and out of the trial, so not everyone who started the study consumed both diets for six years. Moreover, the patients in the FMHS were not randomized, and there were differences between the two groups in blood pressure, cigarette smoking, and use of psychotropic medications. Specifically, among the omega-6 group, fewer subjects were using antipsychotic medications that are toxic to the heart and are known to increase the risk of sudden death. These are the kinds of confounding variables that researchers are *supposed* to control for.

Because the study subjects weren't randomized, the results favoring omega-6 could have been due to the reduction in industrial trans fats in the omega-6 group, or to the increased use of cardiotoxic drugs in the group on the normal diet, or simply just due to chance![47] You could roll dice and have odds about as good for guessing the outcome as you could in trying to ferret out which of the multiple factors at work might be responsible for the reduced deaths from CHD in the omega-6 diet group. One outcome we don't have to guess about: the FMHS is not ironclad proof that consuming more omega-6-rich vegetable oils is good for the heart.

Another study worth looking at is the Los Angeles Veterans Administration Study. This was an eight-year, randomized, double-blind trial in over 800 male veterans with and without previously diagnosed CHD.[48] Researchers compared a conventional diet (with 40 percent of total calories from fat, mainly as animal fat) to an omega-6-enriched diet, in which about two-thirds of the animal fat was replaced by vegetable oils, primarily corn, soybean, safflower, and cottonseed oils. Saturated fat intake in the conventional diet was 18 percent of total calories, compared to just 8 percent in the high-omega-6 diet, and polyunsaturated fat in the conventional diet was just 5 percent of total energy, compared to 16 percent in the omega-6 cohort.

So what happened? Did replacing some of the animal fat in the subjects' diet with vegetable oils make them immune to heart disease? Not really. Subjects who consumed the omega-6-enriched diet saw their cholesterol levels drop by 13 percent, *but this reduction in cholesterol had no significant impact on heart attacks or sudden death.*

There were fewer fatal atherosclerotic events in the omega-6 diet cohort, but this wasn't something the study was specifically designed to look for. It was a secondary, exploratory issue, so the study wasn't crafted to control for confounding factors. Even so, let's not sweep this important finding under the rug and pretend it doesn't exist, the way too many nutrition and health researchers tend to do with facts that may be uncomfortable. Okay, so subjects who ate less saturated fat and more PUFAs experienced fewer atherosclerotic events. Are there any plausible explanations for this besides just the difference in dietary fats?

There are plenty. First, at the beginning of the study, the omega-6 group had fewer smokers overall as well as fewer *heavy* smokers than the conventional diet group: in the omega-6 group, there were 99 nonsmokers versus 86 in the conventional diet group; 38 people who smoked one to two packs a day in the omega-6 group compared to 57 in the conventional; and 7 two-pack-or-more-per-day smokers versus 13 two-pack-a-day smokers in the conventional group.

Considering the extraordinarily harmful effects of smoking on the heart and the entire cardiovascular system, these differences aren't something to take lightly. Second, at the start of the study, the omega-6 group had fewer people who'd already had a heart attack than in the conventional group (327 versus 349, respectively), and fewer subjects suspected of having had a "probable" or "possible" heart attack, as indicated by EKG.

Finally, those in the omega-6 group had almost 10 times greater intake of vitamin E than those in the control group. With a much lower intake of vitamin E in the conventional diet group—an intake the researchers actually called "distinctly deficient"—these subjects were at increased risk for CHD to begin with. Research on vitamin E and heart health indicates that vitamin E may reduce death from heart attacks, so the lower vitamin E intake alone could have been responsible for the higher incidence of CHD among the conventional diet group.[49] Combine that with the conventional diet group having more heavy smokers and more subjects who already had documented evidence of poor heart health? The study was skewed in favor of the omega-6 group from the get-go.

Trans-fat intake was an additional confounder here, just as it was in the Finnish Mental Hospital Study we looked at previously. Trans-fat consumption was restricted in the omega-6 group, but consumption was over 2 grams per day in the control group.[50] Additionally, daily omega-3 intake (as alpha-linolenic acid, ALA) was much higher in the omega-6 group compared to the conventional diet group (about 700 mg/day versus 100 mg/day, respectively). In fact, the control group was found to be overtly deficient in ALA.[51] This study was riddled with shortcomings that might have confounded the results, and it cannot be used as evidence that we should limit our consumption of saturated fats and replace them with high-omega-6 vegetable oils. Another one bites the dust, as they say. *Minnesota Coronary Survey —*

1989   Another very flawed bit of research was the Minnesota Coronary Survey. It ran for four and a half years and was a double-blind, randomized clinical trial involving over 9000 men and women institutionalized in six Minnesota state mental hospitals and one nursing home.[52] (If you're wondering why nutritional intervention studies are sometimes conducted in mental institutions, it's because it's easier to control people's diets that way than when they live at home and may be less than honest about strictly adhering to what researchers tell them to eat.) This trial compared a control diet to a treatment diet that was lower in saturated fat, higher in polyunsaturated fat, and had about the same amount of monounsaturated fat, but less cholesterol. Subjects spent an average of a little over a year on their prescribed diet.

And how'd this turn out? Well, subjects in the treatment group—the one with less saturated fat and more polyunsaturated—saw their cholesterol decrease more than subjects eating the control diet. There were 269 deaths among the men and women in the omega-6 treatment group compared to 248 in the control group; so, a few more deaths in the omega-6 group, but not enough to be considered significant in the research world. There was no increase in cardiovascular risk in men, but women in the omega-6 group saw alarming increases in death from CHD (+28 percent), nonfatal CHD events (+25 percent) and all-cause mortality (+17 percent).[53]

This trial clearly indicates that replacing saturated fat with polyunsaturated fat (mainly in the form of omega-6 from margarine and vegetable oils) is unlikely to reduce cardiovascular risk and may actually *increase* the risk of CHD in women. Moreover, here again we have a study in which cholesterol generally went down, but, at least in women, death from heart disease and from all causes went *up*.

1966 Anti-Coronary Club Trial: ↑ om 6 group → ↑ dths, CHD; ↑↑ a·cause dths

CLINICAL TRIALS WITH DIFFERENT FINDINGS

There have been plenty of clinical trials that have found opposite results to the trials above—but we don't hear so much about those. The Anti-Coronary Club trial found that when saturated fat was replaced with omega-6, there was an increase in deaths from CHD and nearly a quadrupling of deaths from all causes;[54] in fact there was a 71 percent increased risk of death from causes other than CHD in those who replaced saturated fat with omega-6.[55,56] So this study suggests that when you decrease your saturated fat intake and increase your omega-6—exactly what you've been advised to do since the late 1970s—you'll have increased risk from heart disease as well as death from other causes.

—BAD-author shld hv commented on invalidate low sample size

The Rose Corn study ("Corn Oil in Treatment of Ischemic Heart Disease") found that subjects provided corn oil or olive oil had worse health outcomes than the control subjects.[57] Eighty patients with CHD were randomized to one of three diets: a control diet, a diet that restricted animal fat and supplemented with olive oil, and a diet restricted in animal fat and supplemented with corn oil rather than olive oil. By the end of the trial, the proportions of patients remaining alive and free of a fatal or nonfatal second heart attack were 75 percent, 57 percent, and 52 percent in the control, refined olive oil, and corn oil groups, respectively.[58] This was despite the fact that subjects' cholesterol levels were lowered in the corn oil group. That plastic gallon jug of corn oil sitting on the bottom shelf of the supermarket probably seems a lot less appealing now, huh? Let them put it on sale; you don't want it no matter how cheap it is.

Remember, many people who suffer heart attacks or other cardiovascular events have normal or even *low* cholesterol. This cannot be emphasized enough: *lowering cholesterol levels*

does not automatically confer protection against MI or CHD.
So studies that purport to show vegetable oils being better for
heart health than saturated animal fats solely because they
lower people's cholesterol levels are houses of cards that fall
apart easily. If you're wondering why you've spent so many
years using artificially colored and flavored vegetable oil
spreads instead of good ol' butter, you're not alone.

In the Lyon Diet Heart Study (LDHS), among subjects who
had already experienced a heart attack, a Mediterranean diet that
reduced omega-6 resulted in a 70 percent reduction in death and
cardiovascular events compared to a traditional low-fat diet.[59]
That's right: this helpful Mediterranean diet provided *fewer* calories from omega-6 compared to the traditional diet.[60] Intake of
omega-3 ALA was slightly higher in the Mediterranean diet group,
so what the Lyon Diet Heart Study showed was not that a high
omega-6 intake is good for the heart, but rather, reducing the ratio
of omega-6 to omega-3 reduces cardiovascular events and death.
Considering the studies we've already looked at, this next part will
come as no surprise: **all of these benefits occurred without any
significant reduction in cholesterol levels.**

PREDIMED was a large, randomized clinical trial in over 7,400
patients.[61] Two Mediterranean diets were compared with a traditional low-fat diet. The two Med-diets consisted of dietary counseling plus 5 ounces of supplemental extra-virgin olive oil (EVOO)
per day, or dietary counseling and one ounce of nuts—specifically
walnuts, almonds, and hazelnuts. Walnuts are high in LA and
ALA, whereas almonds and hazelnuts are high in MUFA. Thus,
one Med-diet was high in MUFA (from EVOO), and the other was
a combination of increased MUFA from olive oil and omega-6 and
omega-3 from the nuts.

The low-fat diet emphasized reducing all types of fat, including olive oil, nuts, sausages, fatty meats, and fatty fish. Subjects
on the low-fat diet were advised to eat lean meats, low-fat dairy,
cereals, potatoes, pasta, rice, fruits, and vegetables. Compared to
the low-fat diet, the Med-diet + EVOO and the Med-diet + nuts
reduced heart attack, stroke, and death from cardiovascular causes
by 30 percent and 28 percent, respectively. Death from any cause,

not just cardiovascular issues, was slightly lower in the Med-diet + EVOO compared to the low-fat diet.

Subjects on all three diets consumed approximately the same amount of fish and seafood, so differences in intake of the marine omega-3s (EPA and DHA) were most likely not responsible for the benefits seen with the two Med-diets compared to the low-fat diet. Monounsaturated fat was a bit higher in the two Med-diets versus the low-fat diet, but only slightly. Changes in LA intake also don't explain the benefits in the Med-diets, since LA intake decreased in the Med-diet + EVOO, but increased in the Med-diet + nuts; yet both diets showed benefits for heart health and overall mortality.

So what was the protective factor here? The main dietary change that occurred in the Med-diet + EVOO compared to the low-fat control diet was a big reduction in refined-mixed olive oil and an increase in higher quality EVOO. The total intake of EVOO in the Med-diet + EVOO was approximately 50 grams per day (about 1.7 oz.). Similar but less dramatic changes occurred in the Med-diet + nuts group, with a reduction in refined olive oil and an increase in EVOO. In the Med-diet + nuts group, total EVOO intake was around 32 grams per day (1.1 oz.). Compared to the low-fat diet, both Med-diets had substantially greater increases in EVOO intake.

The key takeaway from this study is that complete elimination of refined olive oil and increased intake of better quality EVOO was the factor most likely responsible for the health benefits observed in the two Med-diets. (The Med-diet + nuts group may have also derived benefits from the nuts.) Interestingly, even though the low-fat diet was intended as just that—low fat, but not specifically low in calories—the low-fat group did end up consuming fewer calories than both of the Med diets. Despite being higher in calories, the two Mediterranean diets were better for overall health, and cardiovascular health in particular, than the low-fat diet. Kind of makes you regret passing up a beautiful, fatty piece of traditionally cured prosciutto in favor of a dry, skinless chicken breast.

The benefits of the Med-diet + EVOO group occurred with a linoleic acid intake of exactly 5 percent of total calories—the very bottom of the range some researchers recommend you eat. This study showed that cardiovascular events can be reduced without increasing LA, and cardiovascular events can be *reduced* when LA intake makes up just 5 percent of total calories. So here you have two randomized controlled trials (the Lyon Diet Heart Study and PREDIMED) that tested Mediterranean diets, the results of which do not support the AHA's recommendation that you should get at least 5 percent to 10 percent of your total calories from omega-6 linoleic acid. Hungry for healthy fats? Be generous with the EVOO on your salad, and maybe sprinkle some walnuts on top, too.

Omega-3 Studies

We've spent some time scrutinizing studies related to omega-6 fats. Let's shift over now to the research on omega-3s. Prior to 2005, studies testing marine omega-3s (from fish, or as EPA/DHA supplements) had consistently shown reductions in CHD and overall mortality.[62] However, more recent studies have failed to confirm these findings, muddying the waters and creating confusion among people who want to improve their health. It's troubling that the headlines are so contradictory. We need to get things right here, because this has big implications both for what you eat and how you budget your supplement dollars. Are EPA and DHA good for you, or bad? Does wild-caught salmon deserve its reputation as a "superfood?" It's enough to make you want to give up and head for the nearest fast-food joint. (But don't do that!)

Many of these recent studies suddenly questioning the benefits of omega-3s were plagued by weaknesses and confounding factors, and these shortcomings explain the discrepancies between them and the earlier research. These problems include:[63,64]

1. **Insufficient omega-3 dose used:** If the studies had given higher doses of omega-3 to people who were in need of it, it might have shown benefit.

2. **High intake of omega-6:** Remember, omega-3 and omega-6 fats perform a balancing act; when omega-6 intake is high, more omega-3 is needed to counteract it.

3. **Concurrent medical treatments:** Certain medications or other treatments may interfere with the effects of omega-3 or prevent omega-3s from having the effects they would otherwise have in the absence of those factors.

4. **Too short a follow-up period:** Health doesn't transform magically overnight; changes in fat intake, whether from foods or supplements, may take a while to set in and some studies might simply be too short in duration to account for this.

5. **Lack of statistical power to show benefit:** Studies might have had too few subjects or too few data points to provide accurate and reliable results.

On the other hand, the earlier studies in support of the beneficial effects of EPA and DHA were not compromised by these problems, so let's look at some of them in detail. The Diet and Reinfarction Trial (DART) found that among patients with a history of heart attack, those given advice to increase fatty fish intake had a 29 percent reduction in two-year all-cause mortality compared to those who did not receive such advice.[65] Those who could not tolerate eating fish were given an omega-3 supplement containing EPA and DHA, which reduced all-cause mortality by over 50 percent.[66]

The GISSI-Prevenzione (GISSI-P) trial was a randomized controlled trial testing an EPA/DHA supplement in more than 11,000 patients who had recently experienced a heart attack. Those receiving the supplement had significant reductions in nonfatal second heart attacks, stroke, and death,[67,68] as well as a 30 percent reduction in death from cardiovascular issues, and a 45 percent reduction in sudden cardiac death. The same omega-3 dose was used in another Italian randomized controlled trial (GISSI-Heart Failure), testing omega-3s in nearly 7,000 patients with heart failure. In those receiving the supplement, all-cause mortality as well as hospitalizations for cardiovascular reasons were significantly reduced.[69] That's a pretty impressive track record for some humble fats.

In a Japanese study of more than 18,000 patients with high cholesterol, 1,800 mg of EPA per day reduced the incidence of sudden cardiac death, fatal and nonfatal heart attacks, and nonfatal coronary heart disease events, even when added on top of low-dose statins, which, in theory, should have already reduced the subjects' risk for these outcomes.[70] In a cohort of Japanese patients who'd already experienced a major CHD event or stroke, EPA supplementation led to a 19 percent reduction in major CHD events and a 20 percent reduction in recurrent stroke.[71,72] And remember, this study was done in Japan, where the usual diet is already pretty high in omega-3. The additional omega-3 seemed to benefit heart health *even more*.

DOIT study

In a more recent study, the Diet and Omega-3 Intervention Trial (DOIT), a placebo-controlled trial in over 500 Norwegian men, those receiving an omega-3 supplement (about 2 grams of EPA/DHA per day) showed a 47 percent reduction in all-cause mortality,[73] suggesting that EPA and DHA may reduce mortality in those who have never had a cardiovascular problem—and that even if you haven't had a heart attack, consuming 2–4 grams of EPA/DHA may help you live longer.

Taken as a whole, **research on omega-3s for heart health indicates that these special fats are beneficial for the heart and cardiovascular system in people who have never had a cardiovascular problem, as well as in those who have.**

REAL-DEAL DIETARY ADVICE

Thanks to the 2015 U.S. Dietary Guidelines, industrial seed oils now have their own category as part of a "healthy eating pattern." Currently, all Americans are recommended to consume up to 27 grams of industrial seed oils per day (around 5 teaspoons). This advice will more likely *increase* chronic disease, including heart disease and cancer. We recommend an alternative: our Cyclical Ketogenic Eating Pattern.

A **cyclical ketogenic diet** consists of an initial phase of inducing metabolic flexibility through the use of a low-carb, low-protein, and high-fat diet until one burns ketones, which could vary from two to eight weeks. Once metabolic flexibility is achieved and one has the ability to burn fat as a healthy fuel, then healthy carbohydrates are used in addition to higher protein two to three days per week, typically on days that one is using strength training. Table 1.1 provides a comparison of the recommendations in the 2015 Dietary Guidelines regarding a healthy eating pattern and our recommended alternative based on the data detailed in this chapter.

Table 1.1: 2015 Dietary Guidelines
Healthy Eating Pattern vs. Our Recommended
Cyclical Ketogenic Eating Pattern

2015 Dietary Guidelines Eating Pattern	Our Recommended Cyclical Ketogenic Eating Pattern
Grains, at least half of which are whole grains	Avoid refined grains entirely and even most whole grains; instead, consume more natural, nutrient-dense foods, such as organic grass-fed non-CAFO (concentrated animal-feeding operations) meat, fish, eggs, vegetables, nuts, and seeds.
Vegetables and Fruits	Organic, preferably locally grown vegetables and fruits (the latter in moderation; reach for the more bitter types of fruit, like berries).
Fat-free or low-fat dairy	Consume organic grass-fed non-CAFO animal foods as close to nature as possible, including full-fat or whole-milk dairy products. (Fat-free and low-fat versions often come with added sugar and may increase hunger.)
Protein foods (seafood, lean meats and poultry, eggs, legumes, and nuts, seeds, and soy products)	Consume protein from foods as close to nature as possible (seafood, meat, poultry, eggs, legumes [in moderation], and nuts and seeds); no need to avoid fatty meats. Strive for organic foods and non-CAFO meat, as they will be far lower in toxins and antibiotic-resistant bacteria.

Oils (up to 27 grams/day from olive oil or vegetable oils)	Consume extra-virgin olive oil and avoid industrial seed oils
Consume no more than 10% of total calories from added sugars	Consume no more than 5% of total calories from added sugars
Consume less than 2,300 mg of sodium per day	You need more sodium while on a ketogenic diet. The range of sodium intake that most individuals on a ketogenic diet seem to thrive at resides between 4,000 and 6,000 mg

The American Heart Association does not recommend a specific ratio of omega-6 to omega-3, but as the premier "official" heart-health organization in the U.S., they should; and ideally, it would be no more than 4:1—that is, **your diet should contain no more than four times as much omega-6 as omega-3.**[74]

Additionally, the AHA recommendation to consume 5 to 10 percent of your total calories as linoleic acid should be scrapped and replaced by the far more accurate statement that you need only 0.5 to 2 percent of your total calories as LA. This is sufficient for essential physiological functions, and taking in much more than that might have adverse effects on your health, especially if you consume very little omega-3. The AHA should also specify that omega-6 fats should come from whole foods (such as nuts, seeds, fish, and eggs), rather than from isolated oils extracted from corn, soybeans, cottonseeds, and other industrial sources. Replacing high-LA oils with extra-virgin olive oil would also be a step in the right direction to reduce the risk of cardiovascular events and death.

As the data from Japan showed, even when the usual diet was already high in omega-3, adding additional omega-3 led to reductions in major coronary events. This being the case, the AHA's current recommendation of 500–1,000 mg of EPA/DHA to prevent coronary events probably isn't high enough to provide optimal cardiovascular protection, particularly when Americans' diets are so high in omega-6. A more appropriate EPA/DHA recommendation for the general population would be to consume 2–4 grams per day, especially for those at high risk for CHD and those already living with it.[75] Table 1.2 offers an outline of current AHA recommendations regarding omega-6 and omega-3, and recommendations that are better supported by the scientific evidence.

Table 1.2:
AHA Recommendations regarding
Omega-6 and Omega-3 Intake

[Handwritten margin note: optimal LA = ≤ 2% calories]

[Handwritten margin note left: AHA]

Current AHA Recommendations	Evidence-based Recommendations
[handwritten: !LA = 5–10% cal.] Consume at least 5–10% of total caloric intake as omega-6 . *(LA = linoleic Acid = omg6)*	Linoleic acid as 0.5–2% of total calories is sufficient to support essential biological processes. An upper limit of linoleic acid as 3% of total calories is recommended to prevent enzymatic competition with omega-3 ALA and to reduce the synthesis of pro-inflammatory compounds.[76] If EPA/DHA intake is optimized, then it may be acceptable to exceed this 3% recommended cap. (In any case, linoleic acid should come from whole food sources; see below.)
Consumption of industrial seed oils is promoted	Avoid the consumption of industrial seed oils. Omega-6 should come from nuts, seeds, fish, eggs, poultry, etc.
No advice given regarding the optimal dietary omega-6/3 ratio	Consume an omega-6/3 ratio of no more than 4:1.
Consume 500 mg EPA/DHA per day to prevent heart disease. Those with existing heart disease should consume 1,000 mg EPA/DHA.	Consume anywhere from 2–4 grams of EPA/DHA per day for the primary and secondary prevention of heart disease. However, the consumption of EPA/DHA should be titrated in order to maintain an omega-3 index (EPA + DHA in red blood cells) of at least 8% or more.[77]

[Handwritten margin notes right: ↑ LA competes w. ALA plus ↑ infl; Omb6 : om3 ≤ 4:1; om3 index RBC 7/8%]

Summary

- Saturated fat was inappropriately demonized as the dietary culprit causing heart disease. This was based on the idea that saturated fats raise cholesterol, and the *flawed* theory that higher cholesterol levels increase risk for CHD. The omega-6 fat linoleic acid, found primarily in vegetable and seed oils, with only small amounts occurring in whole, unprocessed foods, was mistakenly anointed as "heart healthy" owing to three *weak* reasons:

  - When people replace saturated fats in their diet with vegetable oils, their total cholesterol and LDL decrease. But remember, this happens only when omega-3 intake is low.

  - Research that included both omega-6 *and* omega-3 has been used to support the idea that omega-6, on its own, is healthy.

  - Higher levels of linoleic acid in the blood are associated with lower CHD risk, but the level of linoleic acid in someone's blood doesn't automatically correspond to the amount of linoleic acid in their diet.

- Industrial seed oils are not nearly as healthy as they're purported to be. In fact, they are actively bad for you, for these reasons:

  - Industrial seed oils were not part of the human diet during the vast majority of our evolution. No population today with good health and longevity consumes them in large amounts.

  - EPA and DHA have consistently been found to reduce the risk of mortality or major cardiac events, *but only when omega-6 intake is low.*

  - Healthy populations, such as in Japan and Italy, typically have an omega-6/3 ratio of 4:1 or less—a ratio easily achieved on a diet of whole, unprocessed foods, but virtually impossible when people consume seed oils and the processed foods that contain them. Recommendations to replace saturated fat with omega-6, especially when it comes from industrial seed oils, have likely *increased* the risk of heart disease and other chronic diseases. It's time to make the vegetable oils vanish and bring back the butter dish.

CHAPTER 2

A DANGEROUS *TRANS*-ITION: THE RISE AND FALL OF TRANS FATS

In Chapter 1, you learned how saturated fats were unfairly blamed for cardiovascular disease. But even with all those flawed studies, how exactly did vegetable oils manage to dethrone the mighty animal fat, a food mankind has consumed for millennia? The story is one of bad science, misinformation, and the devastating consequences of industrial food modification. It's a story that very few know and even fewer tell—but it's one we should never forget.

Our tale begins in the laboratory of Wilhelm Normann, a German chemist. Normann's goal was to find a way to change liquid fats into a more stable and solid form—and his experiments proved to be a success. In 1901, Normann discovered that by using a catalyst and heat and adding hydrogen to liquid vegetable oil, it became a solid. At the time of his experiments, the high demand for animal fats like lard and butter was becoming difficult to meet, and while there was a growing supply of cheap by-product vegetable oils from industrial manufacturing, they were not ideal for cooking. So when Normann figured out how to turn these liquid oils into a shelf-stable, semisolid fat, it was a pretty big deal. Normann guarded his discovery closely, choosing to patent it and share the news with only a few trusted colleagues. Little did he know that his discovery—what we now call trans fats—would set the stage for a global health catastrophe.

In 1910, Procter & Gamble, having purchased the rights to Normann's patent in the U.S., used the technology to create the first commercially available partially hydrogenated fat. We know it as Crisco, and it was hailed as a breakthrough.

The Science behind Trans Fat

Before we dive into the story any further, let's take a moment to discuss what exactly a trans fat is. As you learned earlier in this book, fats are made up largely of carbon atoms and hydrogen in a chain. The specific configuration of this chain will determine whether a fat is *saturated, polyunsaturated, or monounsaturated.* But there are also trans fats, and industrial trans fat is formed when liquid vegetable oil goes through an industrial process called partial hydrogenation, which adds hydrogen atoms to the fatty acids in a random way.

The purpose of hydrogenation is to turn the polyunsaturated fat into a more stable saturated form, which gives it a semisolid appearance and texture. But like many other industrial food processes, there is an unintended consequence: the creation of unnatural fatty acids that your body simply doesn't recognize. **Because the fat you consume later goes on to form the membranes around your body's cells, trans fat can quite literally change *you* from the inside out.** In other words, when you eat food that contains trans fat, the integrity and function of your cells are compromised. Worse yet, trans fat has a considerably long half-life, which means that you'll be stuck with it in your body for a long time. Sure, that blueberry pie with shortening might taste good, but is it worth having trans fat lodged into your brain cells, doing who knows what, for months?

One important thing to note is that there are *natural* trans fats that do not have the same risks as the artificial type. In fact, some research even suggests that the small amounts of cis–trans fat (trans fat whose hydrogen is arranged in an orderly way) found in nature could have health benefits. For example, conjugated linoleic acid (CLA) is a trans fat that is naturally found in grass-fed animals and may have significant cancer-fighting properties.[1] Trans-Vaccenic acid has even been studied for its ability to lower cholesterol levels![2] So, as you can see, the small amounts of natural trans fats found in whole foods aren't harmful and may even be beneficial.

However, the same cannot be said for artificial/industrial trans fat, which can cause cardiovascular disease. How exactly industrial trans fat causes heart disease is not well understood, but a few different theories have been proposed. Research suggests that trans fat can inhibit numerous biological functions, from preventing the synthesis of prostaglandin to inhibiting your body's ability to form long-chain omega-3 fatty acids. Regardless of the exact mechanism, it's a well-established fact that trans fat causes heart disease.[3,4] And there's a growing body of evidence suggesting that its negative effects are even more far-reaching than cardiovascular disease alone; industrial trans fat has also been implicated in diabetes,[5] Alzheimer's disease,[6] cancer,[7,8] neurological disorders,[9,10] and even depression.[11]

But this was not always known. As you're about to find out, industrial trans fat, in the form of partially hydrogenated oil, was very popular through the 1900s.

MARKETING THAT CHANGED THE WORLD'S DIET

The development of Crisco was a success, but there was still one major obstacle Procter & Gamble needed to overcome: how to convince the world to give up time-honored animal fats for a tub of artificial shortening. Their strategy was simple, clever, and deceptive: they would target housewives, who, at the time, performed most of the cooking for their family. Advertisements depicting happy housewives cooking meals for their happy families began popping up in women's magazines. Crisco was touted as a healthy cooking oil and "better than butter."[12]

This marketing ploy went on for decades, making claims that Crisco was digestible, natural, and cheaper. Doctors and scientists were frequently used in the ads, which often insinuated that Crisco would make children grow up to be strong and happy. Strong elements of social influence were also used, with the ads proclaiming that everyone from Grandma to little Johnny prefers pie made with Crisco. They also gave away a free cookbook with 250 recipes that—yes, you guessed it—all used Crisco. In fact, to people at the time, it would seem that there was no reason to choose anything *but* Crisco for cooking and baking.

"...foods so light and delicious that they'll appeal to everybody in the family. Even those who have delicate digestion. Crisco, as your doctor knows, is the pure all-vegetable shortening that is so much lighter!"

— *1938 print advertisement for Crisco*

Procter & Gamble's marketing was a success, with 60 million pounds of Crisco sold in the year 1916 alone. Animal-fat sales began to decline in favor of the partially hydrogenated cottonseed oil. And, for a while, Crisco remained unopposed.

Margarine Enters the Food Supply

Margarine, originally created from beef tallow, found its way into the United States from France in the late 1800s. Initially, margarine wasn't all that popular in the U.S. until manufacturers began to add polyunsaturated vegetable oils to the beef tallow and market it as a healthy butter alternative. This was not met kindly by the butter industry, whose protests resulted in statewide bans and harsh taxes on the production of margarine.[13] According to protestors, margarine was a threat to traditional American dairy farms and butter itself. But despite these bans and heavy taxation, the margarine industry pushed on and adopted the fat hydrogenation process, eventually removing beef tallow in favor of a formula using entirely partially hydrogenated oils.

There was one problem affecting margarine sales: it resembled a pale white chunk of wax. Not exactly the most appetizing appearance. As a solution, margarine manufacturers decided to dye their product yellow—just like butter. The butter industry cried foul and petitioned to block the artificially dyed margarine from entering the food supply. The petition was a success, and for a time, margarine producers were banned from dying their product. Instead, they chose to sell margarine with a packet of artificial yellow dye that would allow consumers to do it themselves. Much to the butter industry's dismay, margarine wasn't going anywhere.

THE DEPRESSION AND WORLD WAR II

The popularity of partially hydrogenated fats grew exponentially during the Great Depression and, later, World War II. The Great Depression, which took place between 1929 to 1939, was an economic crisis that led to worldwide poverty. Many of those who still used animal fats in cooking were forced to switch to the more affordable partially hydrogenated vegetable oils instead.

Things got even worse when World War II began as the need for food conservation became a must. Glycerol, a clear liquid derived from fat, was in high demand for bomb-making, and the U.S. government requested that all households donate their excess fat.[14] **Between the shortages and required rationing, people around the world were forced to rely on partially hydrogenated oil instead of animal fats.**

THE AMERICAN HEART ASSOCIATION JOINS IN

Between marketing, the Great Depression, and World War II, animal fats were down for the count. Procter & Gamble, seeing an opportunity to propel their beloved invention even further into the spotlight, decided they would pay the American Heart Association $1.75 million dollars[15] for an endorsement proclaiming that Crisco was healthier than animal fats.

The American Heart Association accepted, and with that, the demise of animal fats in the American diet was inevitable. The problem with this endorsement by the AHA was that there was no proof of its claim at the time—not a single study demonstrating that natural animal fats posed any harm at all! But animal fats were demonized anyway and booted out of diets around the world. From cakes and cookies to fried foods, the world's demand for Crisco was explosive. Soon, every family had a tub of Crisco in their pantry. Restaurants across the nation used it. And it could be found in nearly all processed and prepackaged foods.

With heart disease rates increasing, the world needed something to blame. During a 1956 nationwide television broadcast sponsored by the American Heart Association, viewers were encouraged to adopt the Prudent Diet, named for its proposed ability to reduce heart disease risk. The Prudent Diet consisted of a torturous regime of cold cereal, corn oil, margarine, and chicken in place of butter, lard, beef, and eggs. Much to the likely dismay of the American Heart Association (and Procter & Gamble), Dr. Dudley White, a participant in the televised show and the personal physician of President Eisenhower, said, "I began my practice as a cardiologist in 1921 and I never saw a heart-attack patient until 1928. Back in the heart-attack-free days before 1920, the fats were butter and lard, and I think that we would all benefit from the kind of diet that we had at a time when no one had ever heard the word corn oil."[16]

But Dr. White later reversed his opinion. President Eisenhower suffered a heart attack, and his doctors sent him home with a prescription for anticoagulant drugs and recommendations to consume a low-fat diet. Dr. White's change of stance, despite the complete lack of evidence linking saturated fat and heart disease, could likely be attributed to his time spent with Ancel Keys, with whom he traveled internationally.

Eisenhower, who ranked rare steak as one of his favorite foods, made it a personal mission to eliminate animal fats and cholesterol from his diet. The American public watched their beloved president's treatment closely, and interest groups didn't waste a minute in broadcasting the fact that Eisenhower was fighting heart disease with partially hydrogenated fats. He died of heart disease 14 years later.

In 1957, a year after the introduction of the Prudent Diet, a researcher by the name of George Christakis decided to put it to the test in a group of men aged 40 to 59. The results of the study showed that men who followed the Prudent Diet had a lower cholesterol level of 220 mg/dl compared to 250 mg/dl of the men who ate animal fats. Christakis was pleased and concluded his study *"appears to have established a reasonable basis for public health action."*[17] That might have been true, except for this buried gem of a statement about the study from a published paper in 1966: *"Eight deaths from heart disease among Prudent Dieter group. None among controls eating eggs every day and meat at every meal."*[18]

Around the same time Eisenhower suffered a heart attack, Ancel Keys was commissioned by the U.S. Public Health Service to investigate the effects of dietary fat. Much like ravenous wolves stalking their prey, the partially hydrogenated fat industry watched closely, eagerly awaiting the perfect opportunity to strike. As we discussed in Chapter 1, the Seven Countries Study performed by Ancel Keys was highly flawed and not at all conclusive, but a study that could link heart disease to animal fat consumption was a huge financial gain for the vegetable oil industry.

Like dominoes, the AHA, the government, and various other health organizations and authorities all fell in line, proclaiming low-fat diets were healthier and safer. Meanwhile, the heart disease rate was steadily increasing, with no end in sight. At this point, it was too late. Critics were silenced, and researchers who spoke out against Keys's crude studies were mocked and had their jobs threatened.

ONE LONE NAYSAYER

In the last chapter, we talked about landmark studies like the Seven Countries Study, the Framingham Study, the Nurses' Health Study, the Finnish Mental Hospital Study, and more—all of which were flawed in numerous ways.

But who was looking at trans fat? After all, organizations like the AHA were touting it as healthier than butter. Where did that claim come from? The truth is, there was little to no science on how trans fat affected the human body, not until 1957. **For the 46 years since Crisco first appeared on the market, there was not a single human clinical study on trans fats. Yet the partially hydrogenated fat industry claimed *their* product was healthier, safer, and better.** If there was no research supporting this claim, does that mean the entire trans fat industry was built on nothing but a far-fetched lie? We'll leave that for you to decide.

There was one very important study that occurred in parallel to Keys's research—before the official gavel came down on animal fats. It was by a biochemist who would later become instrumental in the downfall of trans fats. His name was Fred Kummerow.

At the time, Kummerow was a researcher at the University of Illinois. He managed to acquire autopsy samples from individuals who had died of heart disease. What he discovered was nothing short of astonishing. After examining the samples, he was able to locate artificial trans fat lining the tissue of human hearts. Kummerow published his findings in *Science*,[19] one of the most prestigious academic journals. It was the first published human clinical study on trans fat. You would think that Kummerow's study would have sparked an important discussion and a desire for further research on trans fat. Instead, his findings were met with contempt and he was shunned. But Kummerow was determined to further explore the effects of trans fats, regardless of those who opposed his work. This marked the beginning of his 56-year crusade against trans fats.

Kummerow, who started his day with fried eggs and a glass of milk, was hard at work trying to find a way to convince the world that trans fat wasn't all it was made up to be. By 1968, Kummerow noticed that the heart-disease death rate went up every passing decade. But it was an uphill battle against regulating authorities championing the use of partially hydrogenated fats over animal fats.

Despite this, his research continued though the mid-1970s, when he investigated the effects of dietary trans fat on pigs. The pigs, who were fed artificial trans fat, had deadly levels of plaque in their arteries.[20] Kummerow brought his findings to the FTC, who, shockingly, rejected him because he was a biochemist and not a cardiologist. Then, in 1976, much to Kummerow's dismay, the FDA officially determined there was no evidence suggesting trans fat was dangerous. Worse, Kummerow's efforts to get trans fat banned did not go unnoticed.

Ancel Keys's opinion held great sway with the AHA, the National Institute of Health, and various government policymakers. Keys's power and influence over decision makers may have been the cause of certain researchers losing their funding. Keys did not take kindly to those whose opinion differed from his own, and instead of scientific debate, he resorted to name-calling and public shaming. Among the researchers who lost funding from the NIH was Kummerow. With no other option but to pay his staff out of his own pocket, Kummerow pressed on in his fight against trans fats.

The Tables Begin to Turn

By the 1990s, there was a growing body of evidence that trans fat was dangerous. To defend their product and prove the opposition wrong, the partially-hydrogenated-fat industry spent $1 million funding a study of their own. The results were nothing short of embarrassing. The industry's study, published on October 4, 2001,[21] showed that trans fat actually increased the risk of heart disease more than saturated fat. With the overwhelming amount of evidence against trans fat and the industry's self-incrimination through their own funded study, it would seem trans fat was at its end of days—and yet the FDA did not make a move until 2003.

And instead of outright banning trans fats like Denmark, the FDA chose to enforce labeling requirements beginning in 2006. In short, manufacturers were required to list trans-fat content on the nutritional labels of their food.

To make matters worse, companies did not have to list trans fat content if it was less than .5 grams per serving. This was problematic in two ways. One, most people do not understand how to read nutritional labels. Two, it was still very easy to consume dangerous amounts of trans fat. Initially, the FDA did propose to add a statement to foods containing trans fat that recommended trans fat intake should be as low as possible. However, that was later retracted as the FDA stated they received "very negative comments" about it.[22] It is interesting to note they were more concerned about the trans-fat industry's reaction than the heart disease risk of Americans.

The Downfall of Trans Fat

As research linking trans fat to heart disease grew even more conclusive, Fred Kummerow decided to submit a 3,000-word petition to the FDA in 2009, demanding they ban trans fats. The FDA never responded, despite the strong evidence clearly proving their harm. Finally, in 2013, Kummerow sued the FDA, prompting them to immediately issue a press release announcing a ban on trans fat in the food supply. They did not ban it outright, however, and companies were given a five-year grace period to remove trans fat from foods.

An Important Lesson

Why did the FDA choose to drag their feet in banning trans fat? If they removed it from the American diet immediately, as many other countries chose to do, more lives could have been saved. In fact, experts believe that trans fats are responsible for up to 100,000 deaths per year.[23] If this estimate is correct, the FDA's delay may have resulted in the deaths of millions of Americans—a number that rivals the American soldiers who died in all wars since 1775 combined.[24] And that's just in the last two decades.

How many have lost their lives since 1911, when partially hydrogenated fat was introduced to the market? The death toll could very well add up to one of the greatest disasters in our history. Yet the trans-fat industry and our government are quietly brushing trans fat under the carpet, with many Americans completely unaware of the devastation it caused during its 107-year reign.

It's a lesson that we should all take note of: be careful when you tamper with the food given to us by nature.

Summary

- Artificial or industrial trans fat was created in 1901 to stabilize and solidify vegetable oils, but it had an unforeseen effect: the creation of unnatural fatty acids that your body simply doesn't recognize and that stay in your body, coating your cells, for a *very* long time.

- The trans-fat industry, originating with Crisco and continuing with margarine, convinced the American Heart Association, the National Institutes of Health, and other health organizations that, despite no evidence in the beginning (or, later, deeply flawed "evidence" from Ancel Keys), that trans fats were healthy and animal fats were bad for you.

- With savvy marketing and the onset of the Great Depression and World War II, trans fats rapidly became the primary fat consumption in America.

- One man, Fred Kummerow, stood against the trans-fat industry, as he proved time and again that trans fats were causing heart disease.

- It took until 2003 for the FDA to ban trans fats, likely resulting in the deaths of millions of people.

CHAPTER 3

OMEGA-3 AND OMEGA-6: WHAT'S EVOLUTION GOT TO DO WITH IT?

Back in Chapter 1, we dropped some hints that the abundance of omega-6 fats and the scarcity of omega-3s in the modern food supply are major contributors to the tsunami of chronic disease crashing down on us. If we currently consume too much omega-6 and too little omega-3, how much *should* we be getting, and why? And how did things get so out of balance?

The story of omega-3 and omega-6 is nothing less than the story of *us*—of humans, the diet we evolved on, and its implications for the way we eat now.

It took the entire history of the world to reach a global population of one billion humans by 1850. It took only 80 more years for our numbers to double to two billion in 1930. After that it was less than 50 years until we doubled again to four billion people in

1976, and a mere 10 years beyond that when we tipped the population scales to five billion in 1986. If there's one thing we humans like to do, it's reproduce!

This exponential rise in the human population meant that there was, and still is, a demand for food to be produced ever more quickly and inexpensively in order to feed us. This need for cheaper and faster food was part of what led to the growth and expansion of agriculture, and eventually, to the Industrial Revolution. As we transitioned from our hunter-gatherer origins to settling in locations for the longer term and planting crops—literally and figuratively putting down roots—we began to rely more on grains as a source of calories.[1]

With the advent of industrialization and the mechanization of food production, factories rather than farms became the source for our food. The quality of food was sacrificed in favor of quantity and ease of safe production and distribution. **We have more calories available to us today than ever before, but fewer nutrients. We are, as they say, *overfed but undernourished*.** The three most dramatic changes that occurred with fats in our diet over the past hundred years are:

1. An increase in omega-6, mainly from linoleic acid in industrial seed oils, such as cottonseed, soybean, corn, safflower, and sunflower oils

2. An increase in industrial trans fats

3. A decrease in omega-3 fats—both the type that comes mainly from plants (ALA) and the types that come from animals (EPA and DHA)[2,3]

These changes paralleled the dramatic rise in chronic disease in the United States during the same time period, which is a hint that they are the likely culprits.[4] They're not the only guilty parties, but their fingerprints are all over the scene of the crime. Another important change to our food supply was that we went from eating wild plants to domesticated ones, which are typically grown in enormous monocropping systems—meaning one plant grown in large quantities, with nothing else grown in the same field. Wheat, corn, and soybeans are typically grown this way in the U.S. now, but it wasn't always so.

Perhaps even more important than the change in our cultivation of plants was the change in how we raise animals for food. After evolving for millions of years on wild game and seafood, most meat sold in grocery stores now comes from concentrated animal-feeding operations (CAFO), and increasingly seafood from aquatic farms, which are basically feedlots for fish. Most animals raised for meat, especially beef and pork, start their lives on small farms or ranches, where they eat their natural diet of grass (cattle) or an omnivorous diet (pigs). But when they reach a certain age or size, they're sent to feedlots, where they're fed GMO grains and soybeans loaded with herbicides, in order to fatten them up quickly for market.

These two changes led to significant differences in the nutritional content of the plants and animal foods we now consume. Modern-day plants are lower in omega-3 than wild vegetation was even a few generations ago, and domesticated animals contain more omega-6 and less omega-3 than wild animals and less omega-3 than animals that are grass-fed or allowed to forage on pasture.

The biggest of these changes happened in just the last hundred years. In evolutionary terms, that is barely the blink of an eye. It isn't enough time for humans to have evolved genetic adaptations to do well on this newfangled diet.[5] (Well, maybe a few oddballs among us have. We all have that one friend or relative who prefers highly processed junk food, never exercises, stays up half the night, and does all the other "wrong" things, but appears to be outwardly healthy, looks fit, and could grace the cover of magazines. Unfortunately, those rare individuals are the exceptions, not the rule.) **You are still carrying your prehistoric Paleolithic genes, and these genes are not merely a terrible match for our modern food supply—they are a prescription for absolute disaster.** Your poor DNA has no idea what to do with industrially processed chicken nuggets and baseball-game nachos swimming in "cheez" sauce.

This being the case, if you're looking to restore your health and *stay* healthy into a robust old age, a good place to start would be to return to a way of eating more closely aligned with what your ancient genes are expecting. So what, exactly, is that?

OMEGA-3S IN THE SEAS

From as far back as 3.5 billion years ago until around 500 million years ago, the main form of life on Earth was blue-green algae. There wasn't much oxygen in the atmosphere, so there were few to no organisms that breathed in the way we think of breathing today. However, these algae produce oxygen via photosynthesis,[6] so over time, the concentration of oxygen on Earth increased until eventually it reached a point where new life forms were able to develop. These new life forms consumed the blue-green algae—including the omega-3s contained within them—and these omega-3s became concentrated in the cell membranes of the new life forms.

This is the ancient origin of seafood being high in two particular omega-3 fats, EPA (eicosapenataenoic acid) and DHA (docosahexaenoic acid). Marine life-forms also contain some of the omega-6 linoleic acid (LA), but only very small amounts. Squid, herring, shellfish, and plankton contain as much as 300 times more EPA and DHA than LA, making seafood much richer in omega-3 than omega-6. So omega-3 fats are extremely prevalent in foods from the ocean.

But humans live on land, many living some thousands of miles from an ocean. While populations that lived in coastal areas or on islands would have had easy access to seafood and may have made it a key part of their diets, what about those who lived farther inland? How did humans not living near the sea obtain these special omega-3 fats?

EARLY HUMANS AND THE BRAIN

The way early humans got EPA and DHA when these weren't in their foods is that they *made them* inside themselves. This "biochemical factory" within them allowed them to expand into areas of the world where marine foods were scarce. Since they could synthesize these fats internally, they didn't have to stay in places where seafood was abundant, and this neat biological party trick is still with us today, imprinted in our DNA.

Since you can't make something out of nothing, the EPA and DHA we create inside us have to come from somewhere. They come from the omega-3 fat alpha-linolenic acid (ALA). All humans have the ability to covert ALA to EPA and DHA, but some of us do it better than others. There's no skill or talent involved, so it's not something you can learn to do better. It's genetic.

Brian Peskin advocates for "parent essential oils" (ALA and LA) from plants rather than long-chain omega-3s from fish because most humans don't convert ALA to EPA and DHA very well; he argues that long-chain fats must not be that important for us, and perhaps might even be harmful, since humans aren't able to synthesize them in large quantities.[7] But the process by which we make EPA and DHA from ALA takes a lot of energy. So, during times when our food supply of EPA and DHA was abundant, a limited ability to make this conversion would have been beneficial: we wouldn't have wasted precious biochemical energy on a process that was unnecessary. But when food sources of preformed EPA/DHA were *not* readily available, it would've been advantageous to have an increased ability to convert ALA to EPA and DHA, like an emergency protection mode—something to be called upon when absolutely needed.

All of this suggests that even if—or more likely *because*—some of us have a low ability to convert ALA to EPA and DHA, these special omega-3 fats *are* important for us. And considering that a genetic change resulting in a *better* capacity to convert ALA to EPA and DHA was one of the factors that enabled early humans to expand throughout Africa, it's safe to say that EPA and DHA aren't harmful. Even so, like water and like oxygen, it's possible to get

Expensive Tissue Hypothesis — idea in evolutionary biology

too much of a good thing. So just how much EPA and DHA were included in early man's typical menu?

Over the past few million years, our ancestors' gastrointestinal tracts shifted from being like that of the great apes—a bulky, voluminous large intestine suitable for breaking down vegetables and fruits—toward a system more like that of carnivorous animals: a smaller large intestine not well-suited for large amounts of plant matter, but a highly acidic stomach and a longer small intestine designed to extract nutrients from animal foods.[8] But this change didn't only affect our digestive systems. It also contributed to the development of our more advanced brains. This is an idea in evolutionary biology known as the "expensive tissue hypothesis," and here's how it works: Digestion is a very energy-intensive process. It might not seem like it requires a lot of energy compared to running a marathon, but think about that post-Thanksgiving dinner food coma, when you can barely get off the couch. That sudden lethargy and fatigue have less to do with the tryptophan in the turkey than with all your body's energy being shunted toward your digestive tract and away from your brain. For our hominid ancestors, it took a lot of energy for their intestines to break down massive quantities of tough, fibrous leaves and vegetation.

But over time, as their digestive systems adapted to a diet heavier in animal foods—which are much easier to digest than fibrous plants—their bodies could devote less energy to breaking down food. Fortunately, this energy didn't just disappear. It went toward growing more complex brains—the brains we modern humans have now, capable of composing symphonies, writing novels, and launching satellites into orbit.

They consumed meat from all parts of their prey, including the organs. They cracked open bones and skulls to get at bone marrow and brain.[9] We may cringe at the thought, but ounce for ounce, animal brains contain more DHA than salmon, so unlike squeamish 21st-century folks, early man received ample DHA. Remember that these were wild animals, not ones grown in CAFOs, so the risk of acquiring an infection was much lower than it is today.

Owing to the total fat content of brain, and the DHA content specifically, eating brain tissue would have enabled early humans to support even larger brains themselves, along with a larger body size.[10]

The progression from our prehistoric ancestors to anatomically modern humans *required* DHA, and DHA remains an essential component of our brains today. Remember, fats are essential structural components of all your cells; and DHA in particular is especially abundant in your brain. These days, you get *some* EPA and DHA in your diet, or through conversion from vegetable-sourced ALA, but compared to what your hunter-gatherer genes are adapted to, the amount is miniscule. **The brains of modern humans are about 11 percent smaller than those of humans prior to widespread adoption of agriculture.[11] Our paltry intake of EPA and DHA might be the reason why.**

EVOLUTION OUTSIDE OF AFRICA

The genetic changes responsible for our capacity to make this conversion occurred more than 85,000 years ago—before human migration out of Africa; in fact, the genetic change of an increased ability to convert ALA to EPA and DHA is likely what made it possible for humans to expand their small habitat farther across Africa and then beyond. Some researchers have even called this a "game-changing" event, because it enabled rapid population expansion.

These changes became fixed in those who remained in Africa, but did not remain in populations who settled in what is now Europe and Asia. For reasons we're about to discuss, modern humans in various locations throughout the world vary in their capacity to convert ALA to EPA and DHA. Like we said, we all have this capacity, but it's stronger in some people than in others.

So what happened to early humans who ventured out of Africa? Anthropologists speculate that when our ancestors left Africa, they traveled along the coastlines, spreading across Europe and Asia and eventually crossing into the Americas via a strip of land that, at the time, connected what is now Russia and Alaska.

Staying near the coastlines, their diet would have provided foods rich in EPA and DHA.[12]

Modern-day Europeans and Asians lack the genes to make them good converters of ALA to EPA and DHA. This is the result of their ancestors not *needing* to make this conversion well, since they were the ones who stuck to the coastlines and were eating pre-formed EPA and DHA.[13] The low ability of humans to convert ALA to EPA and DHA persisted throughout the ages, suggesting that EPA and DHA intake during the Paleolithic era was high enough for most of our ancestors that they were able to survive and reproduce without being good "fat converters."[14,15] Unfortunately, the standard American diet is *low* in EPA and DHA, but we still carry the genes of tribes accustomed to consuming high amounts of these. For modern humans, not enough time has passed for genes to adapt and to return to being good converters of ALA to EPA and DHA. For this reason, as discussed in Chapter 1, EPA and DHA should be considered "functionally essential."

Bottom line: just because we *can* make EPA and DHA from ALA doesn't mean we do it well enough to provide our bodies with sufficient amounts of them. We are better served by making sure to get some from our diet or from high-quality supplements.

WILD FOODS

Paleolithic diet authorities S. Boyd Eaton and Melvin Konner noted that the chronic illnesses like heart disease, type 2 diabetes, and cancer as well as mental disturbances like anxiety, depression, and bipolar disorder that plague the Western world today are virtually absent in current-day hunter-gatherers who maintain their traditional diets and ways of life. This is true even for those who reach their 60s, so we can't put this down to hunter-gatherers simply not living long enough to *get* chronic illnesses.[16,17] In the industrialized world, even *children* are being diagnosed with type 2 diabetes, metabolic syndrome, and can become morbidly obese, so these issues have little to do with old age.

Eaton and Konner's research indicates that late-Paleolithic humans consumed around 3,000 calories a day, with 65 percent of that coming from vegetables and the remaining 35 percent coming from wild-game meat. However, a group of researchers led by Loren Cordain, another expert in Paleolithic nutrition, found nearly the opposite. Their study of 229 hunter-gatherer tribes showed that on average, a whopping 68 percent of total calories came from animals with just 32 percent coming from plants.[18] Disparities in these figures may be due to variations in the proportions of plants and animals among tribes living in different locations. For example, those living in warmer climates would have consumed more plant foods; those in colder areas likely consumed more animals. In either case, what's clear is that early humans' diets contained both plants and animals.

Alpha-linolenic acid is highly concentrated in green leafy plants. The omega-3 content from ALA in green plants outweighs the omega-6 by around three to one.[19] For a long period of time, in terms of vegetation on Earth, green leafy plants were the main game in town. The muscle meat of land mammals contains between two and five times as much omega-6 as omega-3, and their fat tissue is closer to being even: about a 1-to-1 ratio. Wild plants have the opposite ratio—more omega-3 than omega-6. About three times as much, in fact. So when looked at as a whole, the omnivorous diet of our Paleolithic ancestors, containing both wild plants and animals, had an omega-6-to-omega-3 ratio of approximately 1-to-1—a perfect balance.[20] But remember: the omega-3 in these plants and animals was in the form of ALA, not the more important longer chains, DHA and EPA, that we obtain from seafood. We mentioned earlier that one of the changes that occurred to our modern food supply—one of the *most* recent, in fact—was the development of CAFOs, where chickens, cattle, and pigs are inhumanely fed heavily contaminated GMO grain-based diets. Cordain's group determined that the ratio of omega-6 to omega-3 in the muscle meat of grain-fed cattle is over twice that of grass-fed cattle.[21] The reason for this is that grains are seeds—and remember, seeds are high in omega-6, while grasses are higher in omega-3. Just like humans, cows are what they eat. When they eat a high-omega-6 diet, their meat and fat become higher in omega-6, and this omega-6 is passed on to us when we eat the meat.

Keep in mind, too, that the reason cattle are fed grain in feedlots is that it fattens them up quickly—much more quickly than if they were eating solely grass, as they are designed to do. Some of the fat they put on winds up inside their muscles— known as marbling, something we tend to look for in a steak, because we all know that fat equals flavor. Meat that comes from grain-fed animals has over twice as much marbling as that from grass-fed animals.[22] Grain-fed animals also have more saturated fat than grass-fed, due to their higher carbohydrate diet. Just as in humans, excess carbohydrate consumption in cattle seems to deposit more saturated fat on their bodies. Bet you never realized how much you had in common with CAFO cattle!

Comparison of Fats from Grain-Fed Animals, Grass-Fed Animals, and Wild Game

- CAFO grain-fed animals have double the omega-6-to-omega-3 ratio of grass-fed animals.

- CAFO grain-fed animals have over twice as much fat marbling as grass-fed animals.

- Wild-game animals have 2 to 4 times more omega-3 than grain-fed animals, and 2 to 3 times more than grass-fed animals.

But if you're not looking for marbling in your own body, you'll want to reduce the amount of omega-6 and increase the omega-3 in your diet. Ditching the seed oils we talked about in Chapter 1 is a good first step, and a good step two would be choosing lifelong grass-fed meats over animals that have spent any time in a CAFO. If you're a hunter or are fortunate enough to have one in your family or circle of friends, you have access to an even more balanced source of these fats. Wild-game meats, such as elk and venison, have two to three times as much omega-3 as grass-fed beef, making wild game a premier source of omega-3s. If wild game isn't an option for you, grass-fed beef, lamb, or bison in moderation are typically healthy options.

$SAD : LA(om6) = 28 grams : ALA(om3) = 1.4 grams$
$Giving\ om6:om3 = 20:1$

MODERN DIET, MODERN DISASTER

NEW

Researchers estimate that the optimal makeup of fats in a healthy human diet should be a 6:1:1 ratio of monounsaturated (MUFA) to polyunsaturated (PUFA) to saturated fats (SFA), respectively. That is, MUFA should be the dominant fat in your diet, with six times less PUFA and SFA. Under the PUFA umbrella, the optimal ratio of omega-6 to omega-3 is suggested as 1:1.[23] How does our current diet stack up against this?

It's believed that during Paleolithic times, total linoleic acid intake (omega-6) was around 7.5 to 14 grams per day, but currently we consume twice this amount.[24,25,26] We have the opposite story with omega-3 alpha-linolenic acid: during the Paleolithic era, we consumed as much as 15 grams a day compared to an almost negligible 1.4 grams today—ten times less. It's even worse for the EPA and DHA. Our current diet contains as much as *143 times less* EPA and DHA (100 to 200mg)[27,28] than Paleolithic humans consumed (660 to 14,250 mg[29,30])—and that our Paleolithic genes still expect.

Brian Peskin has also suggested that supplementing with grams of fish oil causes "fish oil overdose" leading to cancer, heart disease, and diabetes.[31] However, even if you consume high doses of fish oil (around 3,000–4,000 mg of EPA plus DHA per day) this would not be considered an "overdose" when compared to intakes during the Paleolithic times of up to 14,000 mg per day. In fact, what we consider "high-dose" fish oil nowadays actually falls somewhere in the midrange of long-chain omega-3 intake of our Paleolithic ancestors.

With their lower intake of omega-6 and much higher intake of omega-3, your ancestors had a very different ratio of these fats than you likely do today. In looking at total omega-6 to omega-3, the ratio of these fats we evolved on may have been as low as 0.79—but now, we consume as much as 15 to 20 times more omega-6 than omega-3. Aside from being inundated with cheap sugars and refined carbohydrates, this explosion of omega-6 intake from refined seed oils is probably the most dramatic change in our diet since the advent of agriculture. When you look at things this way, it's no wonder so many people are suffering from some type of chronic disease.

Digging a little deeper into linoleic acid, it may not be the overall amount of this omega-6 fat in your diet that's doing the most harm. It could be the *form* it takes. Linoleic acid is an *essential fatty acid*. Recall that when used in a nutritional context, *essential* means that something performs an indispensable biological function, and you can't synthesize it in your body, so you *must* get it from your diet. So it's not that linoleic acid is "bad." You actually require it, but only in small amounts. Things go haywire when you have far too much of it compared to omega-3, and also when the fat is damaged.

There are four main factors that can damage a fat: heat, light, air, and pressure. And the form this damage takes is *oxidation*. Recall from Chapter 1 that oxidation is responsible for causing chemical changes to fats—the fats in your foods as well as the fats in your body. Omega-6 fats, as they were consumed by your ancestors, were protected from oxidation because they remained in their whole-food form—either in animal fats or consumed as nuts, seeds, and other plant sources. This is not how we get our omega-6 today. The vast majority of omega-6 in your diet comes from oils extracted from these seeds, especially corn, soybeans, cottonseeds, and sunflower kernels. During the extraction process, which was only recently created, the fats are exposed to all four damaging elements—heat, light, air, and pressure. So these oils are oxidized during production, and then they're bottled in clear plastic (often toxic) containers that then sit on supermarket shelves where they're exposed to light yet again and continue to catalyze oxidative damage.

New What we end up with when linoleic acid is oxidized is something called *oxidized linoleic acid metabolites,* or OXLAMs for short. OXLAMs have been implicated in causing or worsening many health problems, including chronic pain, cardiovascular disease, and liver and neurodegenerative diseases.[32] You wouldn't want to drive your car across a rusty, rickety bridge where the metals have been oxidized, and you don't want to consume oxidized, damaged fats.

What about saturated fat? Our current intake of saturated fat is around 40 grams a day, which is likely higher than during Paleolithic times. Dairy foods, which were not part of Paleolithic humans' diet, are rich in saturated fat, so that accounts for some of the increase in our modern food supply, and the shift from reliance on wild-game meat to grain-fed feedlot meat has also contributed to the higher saturated fat in our diet. This is a significant change, but you'll see in Table 3.1 that it isn't all that different from the other changes, except for two: **the most substantial changes in the modern food supply are the dramatic reduction in omega-3 intake and the resulting skewing of the omega-6/omega-3 ratio.**

Table 3.1: Comparison of Estimated Dietary Fat Intakes During the Paleolithic Era and the Modern Industrialized Diet

Dietary Fat	Paleolithic Era	Current Day	Change
LA (omega-6)	7.5–14 g[33,34] (None from industrial seed oils)	11–22.5 g/day[35,36] (Almost all from industrial seed oils)	23% decrease up to 3-fold increase
ALA (omega-3)	12–15 g[37,38] (None from industrial seed oils)	1.4 g/day[39] (Mostly from industrial seed oils)	8.5–10-fold decrease
EPA and DHA (omega-3)	660–14,250mg[40,41]	100–200 mg/day[42,43]	3–142-fold decrease
Omega-6/3 ratio	0.79[44]	15–20[45,46]	19–25-fold increase
Saturated Fat	32–39 g[47]	22–55 g[48,49]	1.8-fold decrease up to 1.7-fold increase
Industrial trans fat	0 g	5.4 g[50] (2.6% of calories)	Entirely new in the modern diet; never part of the Paleolithic diet

This table is an estimate of the dietary fatty acid intake per day: "Change" indicates the difference of current-day intake versus the Paleolithic era. For example, there is an 8.5–10.7-fold decrease in ALA intake in the current-day diet compared to that of the Paleolithic era.

Summary

- Humans evolved on diet of leafy green plants and game, with an omega-6-to-omega-3 ratio of around 1:1, and whatever DHA and EPA they weren't able to get in their food, their bodies converted from plant-sourced ALA.

- As early humans ventured out of Africa, they stuck to the shore, where seafood is high in DHA and EPA. Their genes altered with this new diet, resulting in a decreased ability to convert DHA and EPA from ALA.

- Now we eat an omega-6-to-omega-3 ratio of around 20:1. Our bodies are simply not genetically capable of handling this.

- As a result, we are seeing an increase in chronic disease and mental illness.

- With this in mind, the *Superfuel* solution boils down to:

  - Increasing dietary ALA, EPA, and DHA

  - Avoiding industrial seed oils in favor of whole-food sources of omega-6

  - Eliminating industrial trans fats

CHAPTER 4

HEALTHY FATS, HEALTHY PEOPLE: REIN IN THE RUNAWAY OMEGA-6

In the previous chapter, we explored the role of omega-3 and omega-6 fats in human evolution, emphasizing that the Western diet—the one associated with cardiovascular disease, cancer, obesity, type 2 diabetes, and more—is higher in omega-6 and lower in omega-3 than the diet humans evolved on. For nearly the entire time humans have been on this planet, the consumptions of these vital fats were essentially equal. Now, though, our ratio is about 16:1 in favor of omega-6.[1,2]

Besides just this dramatic change in ratio, the total amount of omega-3 EPA and DHA in our diet is *ten times less* than it was in Paleolithic times. As we'll see in this chapter, these changes have had devastating consequences for your health. One of the main reasons why has to do with something that's become a bit of a buzzword in health and nutrition headlines these days: inflammation.

When you hear the word *inflammation*, maybe "flame" comes to mind. And it should. Think of inflammation as a fire in your body. Although a little simplified, this isn't too far off the mark: it's heat, redness, swelling, tenderness, and pain. When you sprain your ankle or get a bad cut, the surrounding area swells, becomes red, tender, and sometimes even warm to the touch; that's inflammation.

Now, inflammation has gotten a bad rap recently, but the truth is it's a natural, necessary process. It's your body's response to trauma. It protects you by keeping damage localized to a small area instead of spreading to your entire body. Without inflammation, you could, in theory, bleed to death from scraping your knee in a bicycle accident.

Inflammation only becomes a problem when it's severe, chronic, and unresolved. This is different from the kind of acute, short-lived inflammation that has important biological value and occurs when you stub a toe or accidentally cut yourself. Chronic, uncontrolled inflammation means that your body is constantly "on fire." It might be limited to a specific type of tissue (like your joints or your skin), or spread throughout your entire body. As with coagulation, where clotting is kept from spreading outside of the damaged area by the resolving process of fibrinolysis, all inflammatory processes need to be properly coordinated with the onset of the resolving processes. There's always a reason for chronic inflammation, though it might not be readily apparent the way a broken arm is. Among other causes, chronic inflammation can result from undiagnosed food allergies or sensitivities, exposure to environmental toxins, or from the cause we're most concerned with here: an imbalance in your dietary fats.

Remember what we said in Chapter 3: fats aren't just the stuff you love to hate on your hips and backsides. Fats are the building blocks for vital signaling molecules in your body—signals that can either help *promote* or help *resolve* inflammation. You might have read somewhere that omega-3s are anti-inflammatory and omega-6s are pro-inflammatory, but that's a bit misleading.

Omega-3 and omega-6 fats can both serve as building blocks for pro- and anti-inflammatory compounds. It's not one or the other. Generally speaking, though, omega-3s produce more anti-inflammatory compounds while omega-6s produce more pro-inflammatory compounds. And since the Western diet is so heavily skewed toward omega-6, many live in a constant state of inflammation, as if their body is constantly awash in damage and injury, but all that's really going on is excessive omega-6 and insufficient omega-3.

So what happens when your body is inundated with arsonist omega-6, without enough omega-3 to put out the fires? Chronic inflammation, which has been linked to rheumatoid arthritis, psoriasis, inflammatory bowel disease, hypertension, atherosclerosis, allergies, cancer, and more.[3]

Populations around the world with a low dietary omega-6-to-omega-3 ratio experience extraordinary health. Whether they live in warm climates or cold ones, in the Arctic or on tropical islands, or have a diet that's predominantly animal foods or predominantly plants, what these healthy groups all have in common is a low omega-6 intake coupled with abundant omega-3. Let's look at some of these in more detail.

GREENLAND

It's been known for decades that Greenland Inuits, a culture whose diet is high in fish and other marine foods, have a low incidence of cardiovascular disease and death from heart disease.[4] Unlike the modern Western diet, the Greenland Inuit diet is higher in omega-3 than omega-6—more than twice as high, actually. Omega-6 accounts for about 2 percent of their total calories, and omega-3 around 5 percent, for a 6-to-3 ratio of just 0.4. Recall that, at 16:1, the ratio in the U.S. is about as far from this as it gets. Between 1974 and 1976, the rate of death from ischemic heart disease among men age 45 to 65 in the U.S. was 40.4 percent, compared to just 5.3 percent in Greenland—eight times less.[5] Cardiovascular disease was also very low in Greenland, causing only

7 percent of all deaths, compared to a whopping 45 percent in the U.S. and Europe.

In Japan, where omega-3 intake is higher than in the U.S. and Europe, but lower than in Greenland, cardiovascular disease as a cause of death was somewhere between the two, at 12 percent. Tellingly, the omega-6-to-omega-3 ratios in tissue samples taken from these populations were 1:1 for Greenland, 12:1 for Japan, and 50:1 for the U.S. and Europe.[6] In other words, the higher the omega-6-to-3 ratio in people's bodies, the higher the rate of death from cardiovascular disease in those populations.

This is due in large part to inflammation and to the effects of omega-6 and omega-3 on blood and blood vessels. After all, the heart is part of the cardiovascular *system*. It's not just things that go wrong with the heart itself that can lead to cardiovascular problems: excessive omega-6 and insufficient omega-3 makes the blood more prone to clotting (which can contribute to heart attacks and strokes), and also makes it harder for blood vessels to dilate.[7] Blood vessels aren't fixed shapes with rigid sides, like the pipes in your home's plumbing system. They're meant to expand and contract—dilate and constrict—in response to your body's variable needs for blood flow. Too much omega-6 and too little omega-3 makes the vessels more apt to tighten and constrict, forcing your heart to work harder to pump blood through them, which can result in high blood pressure, ruptured blood vessels, and other complications.

Greenland Inuits who consume their traditional diet that is naturally high in omega-3s and low in omega-6s live in a very low inflammatory state. So it's no surprise that they typically have low rates of psoriasis, asthma, and other inflammatory conditions.[8,9] Greenland Inuits are also known for their low rates of type 1 diabetes and multiple sclerosis, both of which are autoimmune disorders. Research indicates that omega-3s may be beneficial for other inflammatory and autoimmune conditions, such as inflammatory bowel disease (IBD), rheumatoid arthritis, and psoriasis.

All this information tells us that populations with a low omega-6-to-3 ratio have a low incidence of chronic disease, and when this ratio increases, so does their rate of numerous chronic conditions—including things like psoriasis and rheumatoid arthritis, which can be painful and debilitating, but also cardiovascular disease and type 2 diabetes, which are downright deadly.

(A) Okinawa—Pre 1990—
JAPAN
—Post 1990—↑↑ om₆:om₃

Moving on to Japan, the island of Okinawa is one of the Blue Zones regions and has some of the highest life-expectancy rates in the world. In fact, at one time Okinawans had the highest longevity not just in Japan, but in the world, and they also enjoyed low rates of death from stroke, heart disease, and cancer.[10] Prior to World War II, the Okinawans used animal fats (especially from pork) as their main cooking fat. But by 1990 these healthy and long-lived people had bought into the unfounded fears about saturated fats and were using vegetable oils for most of their cooking. Compared to people in other parts of Japan, who consumed about four times as much omega-6 as omega-3, Okinawans consumed about six or seven times as much omega-6 as omega-3.[11] A Japanese researcher observed that rates of coronary heart disease, pneumonia, bronchitis, and lung cancer all increased as the omega-6-to-3 ratio increased. The saturation of the Okinawan diet with omega-6-heavy vegetable oils and its eclipsing of omega-3 certainly took its toll on the longest living people in the world.[12] By 1990 Okinawan men had dropped from the top spot down to fifth place for longevity among the Japanese. In the same year, while death from all causes in Japanese men over 70 was lowest in Okinawa, in men younger than 50, all-cause mortality was highest in Okinawa. In other words, the older generation—who'd lived most of their lives consuming a low dietary omega-6-to-3 ratio—seemed protected, while those who were younger and had spent more of their lives on a higher omega-6 diet were paying the price with shorter lifespans.

The rest of Japan didn't fare much better. From the early 1900s until about 1950, the omega-6-to-3 ratio in Japan was no more than 3:1. By 1970, it had increased to 4:1, with linoleic acid intake tripling from around 4 grams a day in 1950 to 12 grams a day in 1970. Along with this increase in dietary omega-6 came increases in death from lung, colorectal, breast, prostate, pancreatic, esophageal, and skin cancers.[13]

The increase in death from lung cancer deserves a closer look. There are two main types of lung cancer: squamous cell carcinoma, which is typically due to smoking, and adenocarcinoma, which is not associated with smoking. More than half of lung cancer deaths in Japan are from adenocarcinoma, which suggests that something else besides smoking was increasing lung cancer deaths in Japan after 1950.

Studies in animals indicate that corn oil, which is high in omega-6, promotes lung adenocarcinoma.[14] In fact, high-omega-6 oils in general, not just corn oil, have been shown to promote cancer growth in animals, whereas omega-3 fats seem to inhibit it.[15] Remember, **fats become signaling compounds in your body, and they are also structural parts of your cells. Cells that are constructed with the wrong kinds of fats, coupled with too many pro-inflammatory signals and too few anti-inflammatory ones, may contribute to malfunctioning at the cellular level, potentially resulting in cancer.**[16]

A Japanese researcher summed it up pretty clearly: "Omega-3 fats (ALA in vegetable oils as well as EPA and DHA in fish oils) thus inhibit carcinogenesis whereas linoleic acid and other omega-6 fats are stimulatory [. . .] current levels of LA intake in industrialized countries (6-8% energy) are at saturating levels with respect to cancer-stimulatory activity."[17] This is especially striking considering that, as we saw in chapter 1, the American Heart Association recommends that we get as much as 10% of our total calories from linoleic acid. The Japanese researchers suggest consuming no more than twice as much omega-6 as omega-3,[18] a recommendation precisely in line with our recommendations in this book.

INDIA

Let's journey west from Japan to India. Indian researcher S. L. Malhotra performed a study encompassing more than a million railway workers between the ages of 18 and 55 working in

Healthy Fats, Healthy People: Rein in the Runaway Omega-6

PuFA
(peanut, sesame oil)
Sat fat (dairy)
ghee

different parts of India for five full years, from 1958 through the end of 1962.[19] During the study, more than six times as many railway workers from southern India died from heart disease as those from northern India, and rates of death from heart disease were also low in western and northeastern India.[20,21]

To add to the mystery, it wasn't just the *rates* of death that differed: the average age at death in southern India was *ten years lower* than in the north.[22] Another troubling finding was that contrary to what we would assume based on our understanding of the effects of exercise and general physical activity on health and longevity, mortality was lower among the railway clerks with sedentary jobs compared to the railway workers with physically demanding manual-labor jobs.[23] And when separated by their job categories, mortality was *fifteen times higher* among the manual laborers in southern India than those in the north, even though there were no differences between their ages or the amount of physical labor in their jobs.[24] It's like a detective show: Where's the smoking gun? What's to blame for such a higher death rate in the south than the north?

The researchers ruled out smoking, socioeconomic factors, and stress, having determined that they were not responsible for the dramatic differences in mortality. They also dismissed the total amount of fat in the workers' diets as a contributing factor. In northern India, typical fat consumption was 19 times higher than in the south, yet the rate of heart disease in the north was 7 times *lower.*

These findings were corroborated by additional research published after the railway worker study.[25] Malhotra found that between 1963 and 1964 the incidence of heart attack was over seven times higher in southern India compared to northern India. Again, this wasn't caused by total fat consumption, because Indians in the north consumed as much as 19 times *more fat* than those in the south. The difference was the type of fat. At the time this study was conducted, animal fats, including dairy, made up the majority of dietary fat in northern India, whereas seed oils were favored in the south.[26] In the south, they had a very low fat intake, with most of it coming from peanut and sesame oils.

Contrast this with the north, where fat intake was about 23 percent of total calories, and most of it came from ghee,[27] milk fat, and fermented milk products—mostly saturated animal fats.

Compared to various Mediterranean diets, which are generally 35 to 40 percent of calories from fat, the 23 percent fat diet in northern India is fairly low. But while northern Indians consumed 70 to 190 grams of fat a day, those in the south had an extremely austere diet of just 10 to 30 grams a day.[28] So they may have had a "low-fat diet" up north, but it was high compared to what people were eating in the south, where the rate of death from heart disease was much higher. Malhotra noted that the seed oils favored in the south were about 45 percent polyunsaturated—mostly omega-6— compared to only 2 percent in the animal fats consumed in the north.[29] Up north, Indians enjoyed yogurt, buttermilk, lassi, and other fermented dairy, but this was only a tiny part of the diet in the south.

In the 1950s, death from heart disease was extremely rare in the north of India compared to the Western world. It's one of the lowest rates of death from heart disease ever recorded. Data from India from the 1950s and 1960s show that residents of Delhi, in the north, had exceptionally low rates of coronary artery disease (CAD).[30] In fact, they may have been the lowest in the world.[31] They also had stunningly low rates of other forms of heart disease as well as cerebrovascular disease, which includes stroke. In the 1950s, heart disease in Delhi accounted for 3 percent of all deaths; in Western countries it was as high as 50 percent.[32] At the time, Delhi was a veritable heart-health paradise.

Unfortunately, the detrimental changes that occurred in the Okinawan diet are mirrored in the diet of modern India. As late as the 1970s, India still had a lower incidence of CAD compared to many countries, as well as a low incidence of diabetes.[33] For generations, the main cooking fats in the traditional Indian diet were ghee and coconut oil (which are both high in saturated fat) and rapeseed mustard oil (high in monounsaturated fat and omega-3). What all these fats have in common is a low total amount of omega-6 and a low ratio of omega-6 to omega-3.

By the 1990s, however, almost all the traditional cooking fats in India were replaced with high omega-6 oils due to the promotion of vegetable oils for lowering cholesterol levels. (The U.S. doesn't export just pop culture, unfortunately; it also subjects the rest of the world to its misguided nutritional science.) The Indian diet was always low in EPA and DHA, but it used to be high in the omega-3 ALA (alpha-linolenic acid). Now, however, due to the prevalence of vegetable and seed oils, it's low in ALA and high in omega-6. The balance has shifted from an anti-inflammatory fat intake to a pro-inflammatory one.

These days, the low-fat diet recommended in urban India calls for omega-6 to make up about 7 percent of total calories, and if the Indian guidelines are followed, omega-3 intake ends up being low, leading to an omega-6-to-3 ratio of about 20:1—a massively pro-inflammatory diet. The diet consumed by rural Indians has a 6-to-3 ratio of around 5:1—still high, but a major improvement over 20:1. Compared to urban Indians, rural Indians have a lower prevalence of almost all chronic diseases, especially type 2 diabetes and obesity. The fats consumed by the "health-conscious urban elite" are mostly seed oils that are marketed as "heart-healthy." The result of this is that omega-6 now makes up a whopping 19 percent of total calories, and these individuals are consuming an omega-6-to-3 ratio of about 50:1!

In a more traditional Indian diet—such as that consumed in rural areas—omega-6 accounted for only 5.5 percent of total calories, and the omega-6-to-3 ratio was about 5:1. Approximately 90 percent of this fat came in the form of highly saturated ghee, with the remainder mostly from mustard oil. Researchers noted that on the high-saturated-fat diet, before vegetable and seed oils wrapped their tentacles around the Indian population, Indians had a low prevalence of diabetes. Areas with a higher-omega-6 diet, though, whether in urban or rural regions, had a higher prevalence of diabetes.

The increase in the omega-6-to-3 ratio in the Indian diet paralleled the rise in numerous chronic diseases, but especially type 2 diabetes and obesity. Unlike their famously low rate of type 2 diabetes decades ago, India is now among the nations leading the world in diabetes incidence. In a study in type 2 diabetics, researchers found that reducing total fat intake, *particularly when the omega-6-to-3 ratio was markedly reduced*, improved people's insulin sensitivity and reduced their need for medication to lower blood sugar.[34] Indian researchers know the truth: **"It appears that Indians in chasing the phantom of cholesterol may have lost their rational fat intake pattern and are confronted with epidemics of insulin-resistance disorders. The safety of using omega-6 oils in Indian cooking becomes a matter of serious concern."**[35]

An interesting thing to note about these studies is that it wasn't enough just to supplement with a little bit of fish oil (rich in omega-3 EPA and DHA). The magic wasn't in solely increasing omega-3; it was in reducing omega-6, too, so that the ratio changed dramatically. And this was achieved by substituting vegetable and seed oils with more traditional Indian cooking fats, all of which are lower in omega-6.

KITAVA AND ISRAEL

A team of researchers headed by Staffan Lindeberg, a physician with an interest in nutrition and evolutionary biology, studied a population living on Kitava, part of the Trobriand Islands in Papua New Guinea. The Kitavans eat a high-carb diet: 69 percent of their calories come from carbohydrate, with 10 percent from protein and 21 percent from fat.[36] Their total fat intake is relatively low, but the majority of this is saturated fat from coconut. A minuscule 2 percent of their calories come from monounsaturated fats and another 2 percent from polyunsaturated. The Kitavan diet consists of tubers (yams, sweet potatoes, and taro), fruit, coconut, fish, and vegetables, with negligible amounts of Western food and alcohol. They consume virtually no dairy, refined sugar, grains, or vegetable oils, and relatively little animal fat except for that found in fish, which of course is high in omega-3.

In Kitava, total fat is low but saturated-fat intake is high. In fact, at 17 percent of their total calories, their saturated-fat intake is enough to make the policy makers at the American Heart Association gasp in horror. They consume more saturated fat than is recommended in the U.S., but unlike the modern American diet, the Kitavan diet is extremely low in omega-6 and high in omega-3. Physical activity among the Kitavans is slightly higher than in Western populations, but it's not especially high. Despite high smoking rates in Kitava, stroke and heart disease are virtually absent.[37]

Here again, we have a population with a major risk factor for heart disease—smoking—yet they seem almost immune to it. If you ask the AHA, the smoking combined with their high-saturated-fat intake should make the Kitavans ticking time bombs for cardiovascular diseases. And while they're more physically active than most in the U.S., they're not exactly doing triathlons every day. The deck is stacked against them, yet Lindeberg's group found them to be exceptionally healthy.

Is there now also a Kitavan paradox?

When so many "paradoxes" start popping up, we have to ask ourselves whether these are actually paradoxes—exceptions that don't fit the rule—or if maybe our hypothesis, *our rule*, is wrong. Either saturated fat isn't bad for the heart, excessive omega-6 *is* bad for the heart, omega-3 is protective, *or all three are true.*

Let's now examine Israel's fat experience: if LA (linoleic acid) is good for your heart—so good that the AHA recommends it should make up as much as 10 percent of all the calories in your diet—then you would expect a population with a high LA intake to have exceptionally healthy hearts and blood vessels. But in Israel, you see the exact opposite. Israel has one of the highest intakes of LA, yet the population also has a high incidence of cardiovascular disease and hypertension. Rates of type 2 diabetes and obesity are also high.

Obesity, type 2 diabetes, hypertension, and cardiovascular disease are all driven largely by chronic insulin resistance. There are other factors at work, but chronic insulin resistance is a major player in these conditions. This is also the smoking gun behind metabolic syndrome—a cluster of symptoms diagnosed by three or more of the following: abdominal obesity (a large waist circumference), high blood pressure, elevated fasting blood sugar, low HDL, or high triglycerides. So, with their elevated rates of obesity, type 2 diabetes, and hypertension, Israelis should be on the lookout for metabolic syndrome. And if a high omega-6 diet is suspected to be at the heart of this, what might happen when people reduce their omega-6 intake?

A study from Italy helps us answer this question. Ninety patients with metabolic syndrome were instructed to follow a Mediterranean-style diet, while 90 others followed a "prudent" AHA-style low-fat diet.[38] In the Mediterranean diet, subjects' intake of fruits, vegetables, nuts, whole grains, and olive oil was significantly higher than in the low-fat diet. Their omega-6-to-3 ratio dropped from 11 to 6.7—still high, but a big improvement. People on the low-fat diet had virtually no change in their omega-6-to-3 ratio. Olive oil went up by the equivalent of about an extra tablespoon per day in the Mediterranean diet compared to an almost negligible change in the low-fat group. Omega-3 more than doubled in the Mediterranean group, with almost no change for the low-fat dieters.

So the Mediterranean diet had people eating more total fat, more omega-3, and less omega-6. And what happened? After two years, compared to the low-fat group—which called for a diet that bears an eerie resemblance to the U.S. government's dietary advice (50 to 60 percent carbs; 15 to 20 percent protein; less than 30 percent total fat)—the Mediterranean group had a nearly 50 percent reduction in metabolic syndrome. Despite a higher fat intake, the Mediterranean dieters also lost more weight and had greater reductions in inflammation. And remember, compared to the low-fat diet, the Mediterranean dieters ate more fruit and whole grains, so this wasn't exactly a low-carb diet.[39] This shows once again that obesity and metabolic syndrome aren't solely about carbs. It appears that changing the *fats* in your diet—specifically, reducing omega-6—improves overall metabolic function even without a big reduction in carbohydrates. This doesn't mean it's a great idea to gorge on bread and pasta, but a nice breakfast might be a bowl of full-fat yogurt with some berries and walnuts.

Table 4.1 provides estimates of the dietary omega-6-to-3 ratios of some of the populations we've explored in this chapter.[40]

Table 4.1: Estimated Dietary Omega-6/3 Ratio[41]

Population	Prior to 1960	More recent/current-day
Greenland Inuits	0.4	Unknown
Japan	1–2	4
India (rural)	3–4	5–6.1
India (urban)	3–4	38–50
United Kingdom	10	15
Northern Europe	10	15
United States	7–8	17

INFLAMMATION AND THE OMEGA-3 INDEX

People typically pop an aspirin or an ibuprofen when they have acute pain and inflammation—a headache, a toothache, and menstrual cramps. One of the ways aspirin and ibuprofen work is by reducing the activity of enzymes that promote the formation of inflammatory compounds. EPA and DHA also inhibit these inflammation-causing enzymes.[42] This doesn't mean a few omega-3 pills will magically take away your pain if you accidentally knock your shin into an end table, but it may mean that if you have enough omega-3 in your diet on a regular basis, you could reduce your risk for chronic illnesses that stem from rampant, inappropriate inflammation, such as atherosclerosis, rheumatoid arthritis, and inflammatory bowel disease.

A good way to know whether you're getting enough omega-3 is your *omega-3 index*. The omega-3 index measures the amount of omega-3 fats in your red blood cells. It's expressed as a percentage of the total fats in your cell membranes. An optimal level is 8 percent or above, while below 4 percent is considered seriously deficient. And while we said earlier that the amount of certain fats in your bloodstream isn't always reflective of the amount of those fats in your diet, in the case of omega-3s the correlation is quite reliable.[43] With that in mind, the omega-3 index is typically inversely associated with inflammation: the higher the amount of omega-3s in your red blood cells, the lower their level of inflammation. Let's see how this plays out in your body.

In a study of patients with peripheral artery disease (a condition involving narrowing of the arteries to the legs, stomach, or arms, which reduces blood flow to these areas and causes pain), those with higher omega-3 indexes had lower markers for inflammation than those with lower omega-3 indexes. Indeed, people with an average omega-3 index of 6.8 percent had much lower C-reactive protein levels (a marker of inflammation) than those with omega-3 indexes of 4.5 percent and 3.7 percent.[44] The omega-3 index is also an independent risk factor for coronary heart disease mortality[45]—the lower the omega-3 index, the greater the mortality, and in people with coronary artery disease, the index is inversely correlated with inflammation—lower index, greater inflammation.[46]

INFLAMMATION NATION

The increase in the omega-6-to-3 ratio in the Western diet has paralleled the rise in the incidence of obesity, type 2 diabetes, and cardiovascular disease. Recall from earlier that in general, omega-3 fats are building blocks for anti-inflammatory compounds, while omega-6 fats are building blocks for compounds that are pro-inflammatory. **When you consume a balanced ratio of omega-6-to-3 (1:1 or close to this), your body is able to** keep its normal, healthy, *low level of controlled inflammation in check*—kind of like how the pilot light on your stove is lit all the time, but it doesn't burn the house down. But with so many omega-6 sparks adding fuel to the fire, people who consume a high amount of omega-6 without enough omega-3 are living in a constant state of rampant inflammation, triggering or exacerbating many of the health issues that top the list for causes of death or poor quality of life—cardiovascular disease, type 2 diabetes, obesity, chronic pain, hypertension, autoimmune disorders, and more.

Most government authorities and health agencies recommend an omega-6-to-omega-3 ratio of anywhere between 4 and 19 times as much omega-6 as omega-3. Only at the very bottom of this range do you find a ratio in line with those of the healthy populations looked at in this chapter. Populations with low rates of heart disease, such as the Japanese and Greenland Inuits, have a much lower omega-6-to-3 ratio—about 1 to 4 times more omega-6 than omega-3. As discussed in Chapter 3, this is much closer to what your genes and your biology have come to expect since your ancient ancestors walked the earth. Taken as a whole, the scientific evidence suggests that reducing your consumption of omega-6 and increasing omega-3 is a relatively simple change you can make that will yield profound results for your health.

Summary

- Inflammation has gotten a bad rap, but when it's working properly, it's a necessary, normal body function. Heat and swelling is your body's response to trauma, and it keeps the damage localized to a small area. Inflammation is a problem when it *isn't* working properly; when it's severe, chronic, and unresolved.

- This isn't a hard and fast rule, but essentially, omega-6 fats promote inflammation, and omega-3 fats control it, specifically DHA and EPA.

- By studying the populations of India, Japan, Greenland, Kitava, and Israel, researchers have determined that diets high in saturated fat and omega-3 fat, but low in omega-6 fat, produce lower rates of inflammation, cancer, type 2 diabetes, and heart disease.

CHAPTER 5

DIETARY FATS: WHAT'S GOOD AND WHAT'S BAD FOR HEART HEALTH?

We've spent the previous chapters making the case that as our species has moved further away from the original diet consumed for the vast majority of ancient history, we have developed a major increase in chronic illness. We've looked at populations in very different geographic locations—the Arctic, the Mediterranean, Asia, and the southwestern Pacific—and determined that a unifying factor in their diets, whether they were high-carb or low-carb, mostly plant-based or more animal-based, was a very low intake of omega-6 and a high intake of omega-3. Most of these groups had exceptional health and until recently were largely free of the chronic diseases that have plagued the U.S. for over half a century. As we've seen, though, as these populations have abandoned their traditional diets in favor of what they believed to be healthier—especially for cardiovascular health—they've started to trade their enviable health and longevity for the kind of epidemic illnesses we currently have in the U.S. Thanks to emulating the supposedly evidence-based dietary guidelines created in the U.S. in the late 1970s, almost every industrialized nation now has a high dietary omega-6-to-3 ratio.

Despite a large and growing body of scientific evidence in direct contradiction to those guidelines, recent headlines would like to keep you stuck in a time warp, in a nutritional twilight zone, doomed to repeat the mistakes of the past. With health-food stores well stocked with fish and krill oil supplements, nutrition organizations are suddenly telling you that omega-3s aren't as beneficial as you thought, and that they might even be harmful.

In this chapter, we'll do a deep dive into omega-6 and omega-3 fats as they affect several issues related to cardiovascular health. We'll show you *perception versus reality,* and then look a little further at the role of omega-3 in heart disease before turning to monounsaturated and saturated fats.

Heart Disease

Perception: Regularly consuming vegetable oil lowers cholesterol, and as a result, reduces your risk of heart disease.

Reality: Consuming a large amount of vegetable and industrial seed oils often does decrease total cholesterol and LDL (the poorly named "bad cholesterol"), but *this does not guarantee a life free from heart disease or heart attacks.* If you think having low cholesterol automatically protects you against these, think again. Heart attacks are equal-opportunity killers: they strike people with low cholesterol, high cholesterol, and everything in between.

Just as with fats in your diet, when it comes to cholesterol and risk for heart disease, it's not the total amount, but the type. High vegetable-oil intake increases the small-dense LDL particles that are much more harmful for your heart-health than the large-buoyant ones. It also increases the susceptibility of LDL particles to oxidation, and these damaged particles are much more likely to cause trouble in your blood vessels than ones that aren't oxidized. Finally, a high intake of industrial seed oils often lowers HDL ("good cholesterol"). And if your total cholesterol is lower because your HDL is lower, that's not something to celebrate.

THE ROLE OF OMEGA-3

Perception: Omega-3 fats (EPA and DHA) may increase LDL and therefore increase your risk of heart disease. Additionally, omega-3s may raise your blood sugar and insulin levels and are inherently susceptible to oxidation and thus may increase oxidative damage in your body.

Reality: It's true that EPA and DHA can increase LDL, but unlike the omega-6 seed oils, they tend to increase the benign large-buoyant type while reducing the more harmful small-dense type—the type more likely to build up inside your artery walls. So the overall influence of EPA and DHA on LDL is beneficial. Additionally, EPA and DHA reduce inflammation and the tendency for your blood to form dangerous clots—such as those that can cause a heart attack and stroke. These important fats can also reduce blood pressure and improve the overall health and function of your blood vessels—the dilating and constricting discussed in Chapter 4.

The reason recent studies have started to question the benefits of omega-3s is that in some circumstances, they haven't shown the positive impact expected from them. What were those circumstances? High omega-6 intake! Studies involving omega-3 supplementation often fail to take into account a person's typical diet. If their usual diet—the typical Western diet—is flooded with an ocean of omega-6, then throwing a little splash of omega-3 in it isn't going to make much difference. On the other hand, when someone's diet is relatively low in omega-6, or when the research looks at the ratio of omega-3 fatty acids in tissues, EPA and DHA have consistently been found to be helpful for cardiovascular health.

BLOOD PRESSURE

Perception: Marine omega-3 fats (EPA and DHA) do not have any benefit for lowering blood pressure. Omega-6 seed oils do not raise blood pressure.

Reality: Consuming EPA and DHA, especially in combined doses of 3 grams or more per day, has been found to significantly reduce blood pressure, particularly in patients with diabetes or heart disease. Consuming omega-6 seed oils may increase blood pressure and damage healthy arteries.

High blood pressure, called *hypertension*, is referred to as "the silent killer." The reason for this is that in many people, it comes with no warning signs or symptoms. Unlike other cardiovascular problems, which may cause chest pain, shortness of breath, or other symptoms, hypertension takes hold and progresses quietly, even while it's causing damage to the heart and blood vessels. Because it's so insidious, it's something you really want to keep an eye on. With that in mind, let's look at the roles of different factors in helping to maintain healthy blood pressure.

SALT

Perception: The dietary villain that has traditionally borne the blame for causing hypertension is salt, which is said to cause the body to retain water, putting stress on the heart and blood vessels.

Reality: Healthy people have been consuming salt since the dawn of time. It is an innocent victim in the blood-pressure game—while omega-6 fats have been largely ignored, though they are *far more* detrimental for blood pressure than sodium. (Dr. DiNicolantonio's book *The Salt Fix* provides powerful arguments that salt—which has been prized and valued throughout history—is not the primary cause of high blood pressure. In fact, a diet that's too *low* in sodium can actually cause your blood pressure to rise.)

FAT

Perception: Eating fats gives you clogged arteries.

Reality: If you have a typical view of nutrition, you are likely unaware of the true effect of fats on your arteries. Proper blood-vessel function is controlled by compounds that help your vessels dilate and constrict in response to blood flow—and the vessels *must* dilate. If they don't, blood has a harder time flowing through them, and your blood pressure will rise.

One of the primary compounds that helps your blood vessels dilate is *nitric oxide.* (Don't confuse this with nitrous oxide, the "laughing gas" used in dentist's offices.) Besides just telling your arteries to dilate, nitric oxide can also help prevent clots and atherosclerotic plaques from forming.[1] All of that sounds good so far. Where do the fats come in?

As we've discussed, omega-6 fats such as linoleic acid are highly susceptible to oxidation. Oxidized, damaged linoleic acid sets off a cascade that ends with reducing the synthesis of nitric oxide.[2] Less nitric oxide, higher blood pressure.[3]

Additionally, recall that a high intake of omega-6 fats increases small-dense LDL and also oxidized LDL. Oxidized LDL is found in the plaques that build up in artery walls,[4] and the plaques may interfere with proper blood-vessel function. Adding insult to arterial injury, omega-6 fats don't just affect your blood pressure by interfering with your blood vessels' ability to dilate. They may also promote the formation of compounds that actively direct your blood vessels to constrict.[5] Soybean, corn, and cottonseed oils start looking much less "heart-healthy" when you know they contribute to atherosclerosis and hypertension.[6] However, this does not necessarily apply to omega-6 found in its natural food state such as in nuts and seeds.

Figure 5.1 compares the old and new dogmas regarding the role of linoleic acid in coronary heart disease.

OLD dogma:

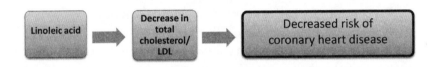

NEW dogma:

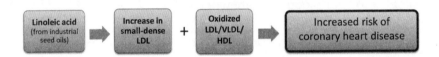

Figure 5.1: Old and new dogma regarding omega-6 linoleic acid and risk for CHD

FATS AND BLOOD PRESSURE

Let's start with the ones we know best at this point. How do omega-3 fats stack up against omega-6 with regard to blood pressure? One study showed that in people with mild hypertension, taking 6 grams of fish oil a day for 10 weeks lowered blood pressure compared to 6 grams of corn oil.[7] In fact, the corn oil actually *increased* arterial pressure, although only by a little bit.[8] But when your blood pressure is already elevated, something that makes it even slightly higher could tip you from a category where you don't need medication into one where you do. At the very least, fish oil appears to be better than omega-6-rich corn oil for lowering your blood pressure, and the beneficial effects can be seen in as little as 10 weeks. Now, 6 grams of long-chain omega-3s is a relatively high dose, but that amount of total omega-3 is easily obtainable on a healthy diet that contains abundant marine omega-3-rich foods, with a little extra supplementation.

So EPA and DHA are better for blood pressure than corn oil. But what about other kinds of fat? How about monounsaturated fat? Does omega-6 have an edge there, or does it still fail to impress?

In a study that pitted olive oil (high monounsaturated) against sunflower oil (high omega-6) in people with high blood pressure, olive oil was the clear winner. For six months, people consumed a diet high in monounsaturated fat and low in polyunsaturated or a diet lower in monounsaturated fat and higher in polyunsaturated.[9] After six months, they switched over to the other diet, so that the effects of both diets could be evaluated in all participants.

So, how good was the sunflower oil for heart health? Not as good as the American Heart Association would like you to believe. Remember, they recommend that you get as much as 10 percent of your calories from omega-6. The sunflower-oil diet was right in that ballpark. Study participants started out with an average blood pressure of 134/90 mmHg (normal is less than 120/80 mmHg).[10] At the end of the olive-oil diet, their average blood pressure had *decreased* to 127/84 mmHg—still slightly elevated, but much closer to healthy. After the sunflower-oil diet, blood pressure didn't drop at all—in fact, it slightly increased to 135/90 mmHg.

The real kicker, though, was in people's medication. After the olive-oil diet, study participants' blood pressure medication was reduced by 48 percent, compared to just 4 percent after the sunflower-oil diet. Eight on the olive-oil diet were able to quit their medication altogether, while all on the sunflower oil continued to require medication. Not only that, but two people who didn't need blood-pressure medication at the start of the sunflower-oil diet *did* need it afterward! The researchers believed that besides differing effects of the various fatty acids in the two oils, the polyphenols in the olive oil likely increased nitric oxide, which would have resulted in lower blood pressure.[11] Polyphenols are responsible for the peppery bite some olive oils have, or the mild burning sensation you feel at the back of your throat when you taste a high-quality olive oil. So if you enjoy sunflower seeds, it's okay to eat them occasionally in your salad or at a ballgame (although some physicians like Steven Gundry believe most seeds should be avoided due to their high lectin content), but you need to avoid using seed oils when you cook.

The list below summarizes potential mechanisms by which the omega-6 fat linoleic acid contributes to hypertension:

- May reduce synthesis of nitric oxide[12]
- Inhibits insulin signaling and eNOS activation in the vasculature[13]
- Increases oxidized LDL, which may result in blood-vessel dysfunction and hypertension[14]
- Increased production of compounds that constrict blood vessels[15]
- Increase in chronic inflammation, resulting in blood-vessel dysfunction[16,17]

THE BENEFITS OF EPA AND DHA

High doses of marine omega-3 fats have natural blood-thinning properties. This is a major benefit if you are at risk for conditions involving blood that is hypercoagulable—that is, blood that forms clots too easily. People with metabolic syndrome, which results primarily from insulin resistance, often have hypercoagulable blood.[18] As you'll recall from the previous chapter, a high intake of omega-6 fats seems to contribute to insulin resistance. Think of it this way: when insulin resistance is present, especially when blood sugar is also high, instead of smooth and fluid water that flows through blood vessels easily, blood becomes more like a thick sludge pressing up against your arteries. No wonder your blood pressure goes up.

In a study of obese individuals with hypertension and poor blood-lipid profiles, supplementing with fish oil led to lower blood pressure and triglycerides, and a normalization of blood clotting.[19] In another study involving both nondiabetics and those with type 2 diabetes, fish-oil supplementation resulted in impressive reductions in systolic blood pressure (the top number). Nondiabetics went from an average systolic pressure of 159 to 146 mmHg; diabetics' average systolic pressure dropped from 158 to 142 mmHg. Even with these dramatic reductions, these individuals were still hypertensive, but marine oil certainly helped things start to trend in a much healthier direction. Fish oil is powerful stuff, but we can't expect it to do *everything*. Combined with other dietary and lifestyle interventions, blood pressure would likely come down even further.

Research that analyzed the findings of 31 studies that compared fish oil to a placebo found that fish-oil supplementation causes a dose-dependent reduction in blood pressure—meaning, the higher the dose of fish oil, the greater the reduction in blood pressure.[20] We should note, though, that the greatest effects were seen when people took at least 3.3 grams of fish oil a day, and the results were strongest in people with hypertension, abnormal lipid profiles, and atherosclerosis.

This makes sense, though: **if your heart and blood vessels are already in great shape, and your blood pressure is already at a healthy level, then fish oil might not do all that much for you.** But if you're starting from a place of high blood pressure or have other cardiovascular issues, fish oil or krill oil may be a natural way to help yourself. Another analysis of several trials backs this up: when given at doses above 3 grams per day, long-chain omega-3 fats reduced blood pressure only by an almost negligible amount in people with normal blood pressure, but the reduction was notably greater in those with high blood pressure.[21]

Other studies corroborate these findings. An analysis of 36 randomized trials found that an average dose of 3.7 grams of fish oil per day causes significant reductions in blood pressure.[22] Another analysis of 16 trials showed that omega-3 supplementation (ranging from 0.5 to 4.5 grams per day over an average of about two months) improved blood-vessel dilation.[23] These results were confirmed in those who were overweight or had type 2 diabetes.[24] Cardiovascular problems are the leading cause of death among type 2 diabetics, so an intervention that leads to better heart and blood-vessel function are most welcome in this population—especially when it's something as simple and inexpensive as taking fish or krill oil.

ALA: The "Parent" Omega-3

Recall from the introduction that alpha-linolenic acid (ALA) is considered the "parent" omega-3 and linoleic acid (LA) is considered the "parent" omega-6 because these are the starting compounds that can be converted into other kinds of omega-3 and omega-6 fats. If you think of a family tree, with many branches of children and relatives coming down from two parents at the top, ALA and LA are at the top of the omega-3 and omega-6 fatty-acid family trees.

ALA, found in leafy greens, flaxseeds, walnuts, and some legumes, is the parent compound whose offspring are EPA and DHA. We've explained that through our adaptation to different geographic habitats and food supplies, most of us have a very limited ability to convert ALA into EPA and DHA, and are better served by getting these fats preformed from seafood. Nevertheless, ALA itself, independent of EPA and DHA, seems to have beneficial effects on blood pressure.

One study showed that for each 1 percent increase in the amount of ALA in stored body fat, there was a decrease of 5 mmHg in systolic and diastolic blood pressure.[25] Again, 5 points might not sound like much, but with current diagnostic standards, even a one- or two-point change could mean the difference between officially being diagnosed with hypertension and receiving medication—which typically comes with unpleasant and sometimes dangerous side effects—or staying in a less risky category, with your doctor more likely recommending diet and lifestyle changes.

To reduce your risk for "the silent killer," ensure you have an adequate intake of omega-3 fats and reduce your consumption of omega-6. If you're already living with high blood pressure or cardiovascular disease, you'll want to optimize your balance of these fats. We'll show you how to do this in Chapter 8. In the meantime, let's pivot from blood pressure to lipids—the fats and cholesterol in your blood.

BLOOD LIPIDS

Much of the confusion surrounding dietary fats—the good, the bad, and the deadly—has to do with the effects that different fats found in your *food* has on the fats found in your *blood*. Here, we'll cover the best available scientific evidence to help you separate good fats from bad fats when it comes to blood fats—which we call lipids.

Saturated fat and, to a lesser degree, omega-3 fat have been demonized as contributing to heart disease because they typically raise LDL. Conversely, vegetable and seed oils, which are high in omega-6, have been celebrated as healthy for their ability to lower cholesterol. However, as previously explored, looking solely at total cholesterol or LDL has led us astray in trying to identify which fats we should welcome into our diet and which ones we should kick out.

A study done in the U.K. looked at four different diets, all of which had polyunsaturated fats making up about 6 percent of the total calories. Where they differed was in the amount of omega-6 and omega-3. A diet that had an omega-6-to-3 ratio of 3:1—close to what we evolved on—led to improvements in blood lipids that were not seen in a diet that had an omega-6-to-3 ratio of 11:1. Reducing the omega-6-to-3 ratio increased LDL particle size and also increased HDL, both of which are beneficial for cardiovascular health.[26]

Another study, one that had participants from multiple centers across Europe, showed that certain fats were beneficial for the lipid profile in those with metabolic syndrome.[27] A diet high in monounsaturated fat and a low-fat diet that contained extra omega-3s helped shift people from "pattern B" to "pattern A" lipoproteins—that is, from the harmful small-dense to the benign large-buoyant LDL—when compared to a diet high in saturated fat and a low-fat diet that contained sunflower oil. Triglycerides were also lowered in both of these groups (elevated triglycerides are a marker for increased cardiovascular disease).[28]

Recall that LDL, per se, isn't harmful. It's really the small-dense LDL particles that tend to get you into trouble, and even more so, *oxidized* LDL particles. In a study of people with familial hyperlipidemia (genetically very high cholesterol), omega-3 supplementation (3.4 grams of EPA and DHA) lowered triglycerides by over 25 percent in just eight weeks—*not bad.*[29] Their LDL went up by 21 percent, but the increase was primarily due to a greater number of the large-buoyant type, and there was a reduction in the small-dense type. So omega-3 led to an increase in the total amount of LDL, but the pattern shifted to one that's better for cardiovascular health.[30] At least seven trials have found that omega-3s increase LDL particle size or shift LDL from pattern B (bad) to pattern A (good).[31] Conventional medicine needs to stop looking at LDL as the bad guy. Like so much in health and nutrition, it's just not that simple.

Let's look at a study where men with poor lipid profiles followed one of three diets: one enriched with flaxseed oil (high in the omega-3 ALA), one enriched with sunflower oil (high in omega-6), or one enriched with sunflower oil plus fish oil (high in the long-chain omega-3s EPA and DHA). After 12 weeks on their diets, men in all three groups had lower cholesterol levels than when they started.[32] However, triglycerides came down only in the men in the flax- and fish-oil groups, not those in the sunflower-oil group. In another change you can hang your hat on by now, the fish-oil group had a reduction in small-dense LDL and an increase in HDL. With a decrease in triglycerides coupled with an increase in HDL, the men in the fish-oil group saw a substantial improvement in their risk for coronary heart disease. This ratio—triglycerides-to-HDL—is a better predictor of CHD than LDL.

It's worth noting that some of the benefits observed in the fish-oil group, such as an increase in HDL and a decrease in small-dense LDL, were not seen in the flax-oil group. So even though flax oil is high in omega-3 from alpha-linolenic acid (ALA), EPA and DHA are more powerful when it comes to improving markers for heart health. The improvements seen in the men in the fish-oil group seemed to correlate with higher amounts of DHA in their tissue.[33]

DHA vs. EPA for Blood Lipids

When it comes to improving blood lipids, it appears there's something unique about EPA and DHA that's not found in ALA. So to improve your lipid profile, it might not be enough to simply increase ALA, commonly referred to as plant omega-3s, in general. You might need to be more specific by consuming EPA and DHA. But which? Both? Let's take a closer look at this.

The improvements in LDL size and density seem to be due mostly to DHA, rather than EPA.[34,35] In a study of healthy people with normal cholesterol, HDL levels increased by 13 percent when subjects took 2.3 grams of DHA per day, but not when they took about the same amount of EPA.[36] DHA is also better than EPA for reducing triglycerides.[37] In patients with abnormal lipids, 3 grams of DHA per day reduced triglyceride levels more than the same amount of EPA.[38] Independently of EPA, DHA also seems to have protective effects against cardiac arrhythmias (an abnormal heartbeat), clotting, and arterial plaque formation.[39]

This may seem like a moot point, because the fact is, unless you have access to highly processed oils, it's almost impossible to get pure EPA or pure DHA. As they occur naturally in foods, they're typically found together. Most omega-3 supplements also contain both, though they usually have a little more EPA than DHA. But some brands are higher in DHA than others, and this might be beneficial if you're looking to take advantage of some of the specific properties that DHA has to offer.

Platelets and Coagulation

Platelets are the cells in your blood responsible for coagulation—for forming clots. At first glance, blood clots sound like a bad thing. After all, blood clots are big players in heart attacks and strokes, and if a clot breaks away from a blood vessel and travels to the lungs, it can actually be deadly—that's a pulmonary embolism. But not all clotting is bad. Just as with inflammation, clotting is a natural, normal, lifesaving process—one that can keep you from bleeding to death—as long as it happens where and when it's supposed to. The trouble comes when the blood becomes too viscous and thick, and prone to excessive clotting. Drugs referred to as "blood thinners" are designed to help people whose blood clots too easily, which puts them at risk for strokes, heart attacks, and pulmonary embolism.

It's been known for quite some time that EPA and DHA are natural blood thinners; high-dose EPA and DHA might even work like patented pharmaceuticals do, but with fewer side effects. EPA and DHA are both effective for this, but as we saw with effects on cholesterol and other lipids, DHA has a slight edge over EPA for reducing platelet aggregation—the formal term for clotting.

But what if you don't like popping so many pills? Most EPA and DHA capsules are large, so maybe you don't like swallowing them, or maybe you'd simply prefer to get your EPA and DHA the old-fashioned way—from healthy fish. If so, you're in luck. Fatty fish does the trick. In people who consumed a little over a pound of oily fish per week for just four weeks, markers for platelet aggregation were reduced by 35 percent compared to those people who didn't eat that much fish, and the markers went back to their previous values after the fish consumption stopped.[40]

This makes sense. **Your body is a dynamic, ever-changing biochemical system. If you want to experience the positive effects of something, you have to *keep doing* the things that created those effects.** If you want healthy teeth and gums, you can't just brush your teeth once and never do it again; you have to keep the habit up. It's the same with healthy fats, whether you get them from whole foods or from supplements. You can't expect to continue reaping the benefits of omega-3s if you eat fish for dinner one evening and never have it again, or take EPA and DHA for a week but then forget about it after that.

If blood clotting is a normal, natural process, is it possible to have too *little* clotting? We know that too much clotting can be a disaster, but can you take so much omega-3 that your blood doesn't clot *enough?* Thick, viscous blood is hard for the heart to pump, but what if your blood gets too thin? This seems to be an unfounded fear. A researcher who looked into this issue found that patients who had been supplementing with omega-3s prior to major surgeries had a "virtually nonexistent" risk for significant bleeding.[41] Women sometimes lose a great deal of blood during childbirth, for instance, but one study found that pregnant women who had consumed about 2.7 grams of omega-3 daily did not have increased blood loss during delivery.[42]

One group of people who might want to be careful with omega-3 supplementation are those already taking blood-thinning or anticoagulant medications. If you're already taking a powerful drug to thin your blood, thinning it even more could have undesirable effects—that just makes logical sense. But the fact is that evidence indicates that even for these people, omega-3 supplements don't increase the risk for bleeding problems.[43]

The following are beneficial effects of EPA and DHA on lipids. In all cases, DHA is more potent than EPA, but that's not to malign EPA or make it sound unimportant. EPA has other positive effects outside the cardiovascular system, so you shouldn't avoid EPA. It just means that if you're looking for a good EPA *and* DHA supplement, you might do best to look for one that's high in DHA. (We'll show you how to choose appropriate supplements in Chapter 8.)

The benefits of EPA and DHA on lipids and platelets include:

- Reduced triglycerides
- Reduced small-dense LDL
- Increased large-buoyant LDL
- Increased HDL
- Optimized platelet aggregation (excessive clotting)

Heart Attack and Sudden Cardiac Death

The most common symptom of heart disease is, unfortunately, sudden death, as it is responsible for 50 percent to 60 percent of all deaths from coronary artery disease,[44] which is why it is vital to have a proactive approach. Most people with heart disease don't get a second chance.

Around 300,000 people in the U.S. die every year from non-traumatic out-of-hospital sudden cardiac arrest—that is, their heart stops without warning and it doesn't start again. Many of these cases are caused by abnormal heart-muscle contraction (called fibrillation) due to clotting.[45,46] EPA and DHA may be one of the best strategies for reducing this risk. Studies suggest that if your intake of omega-3 is low, especially if it's combined with a high intake of omega-6, you're at greater risk not only of having a heart attack but also of *dying* from one. In a study out of Italy, patients who supplemented with EPA and DHA after a heart attack had a lower rate of sudden cardiac death within four months.[47]

In 2003 the European Society of Cardiology recommended that fish oil be part of standard patient treatment after a heart attack.[48] In fact, it's been shown that just three months of fish oil supplementation can reduce mortality after a heart attack.[49] Evidence from many trials indicates that fish or fish oil reduce cardiovascular mortality from 30 percent to 50 percent and may reduce sudden cardiac death as much as 45 percent to 81 percent.[50] If a pharmaceutical company could develop a drug with those kinds of benefits, it would be a gold mine that would no doubt cost you a fortune to refill at the local pharmacy. But lucky for you, you can head to a health-food store and get these same benefits with a good-quality EPA and DHA supplement.

The incidence of sudden cardiac death in the general population of Western countries is almost twenty times greater than that in Japan,[51] as the omega-3 index strikes again. The average omega-3 index in Japan is about 10 percent, compared to just 4.5 percent in Western countries.[52,53] **An omega-3 index of 8 percent or higher is associated with a 90 percent reduction in the risk of sudden cardiac death compared to an index of 4 percent**

or less.[54] Put differently, people with an omega-3 index below 4 percent have a risk of sudden cardiac death ten times greater than those whose index is above 8 percent.[55] People with an omega-3 index of 5 percent have a 70 percent lower risk of cardiac arrest compared to people at 3 percent,[56] so inching your index higher is certainly beneficial—but we can do better. For most of us, getting our index closer to 10 percent (as is found in Japan) might provide the biggest benefit for cardiovascular health.

As you can see, the omega-3 index is a vital piece of information that will help you optimize your balance of EPA and DHA. Sadly, it is not available at most commercial labs like Quest or LabCorp, but there are specialty labs that will do the test relatively inexpensively and conveniently. There is no need to go to a lab: you merely request a kit, and once you receive it in the mail, you take a few drops of blood from your fingertip and apply it to a blotter card and mail it back to the lab. If you are interested in this test you can go to www.mercola.com/omega3test.

CORONARY HEART DISEASE

Southern Europeans, such as Greeks from Crete, are known for their low rates of cardiovascular disease. Compared to Northern Europeans—who have higher rates of heart disease—their diets are higher in monounsaturated fat (mostly from olive oil) and lower in omega-6 fat.[57]

The primary type of fat in olive oil, called oleic acid, has been found to have multiple positive effects on cardiovascular health: it reduces the susceptibility of LDL to oxidation, reduces blood coagulation, and improves blood-vessel function.[58]

Epidemiologically, a high intake of oleic acid, as in the Mediterranean diet, is correlated with a low rate of heart disease, while a high intake of omega-6 from vegetable oils is correlated with a *high* rate not only of heart disease but also high blood pressure, type 2 diabetes, and obesity.[59,60,61] The most recent incarnation of the U.S. dietary guidelines, from 2015, recommends the consumption of "oils," which include olive oil *or* high-omega-6 vegetable oils, with no details on which might be preferable—perhaps that is better than not recommending olive oil at all, but as we've covered, there are many lines of evidence that suggest that olive oil (especially high-quality extra-virgin olive oil) is good for your heart, while omega-6-rich oils are anything but.

EXTRA-VIRGIN OLIVE OIL: GOING THE EXTRA MILE

It is commonly believed that extra-virgin olive oil, especially when compared to refined olive oil, is healthier due to its higher polyphenol content. One trial sought to determine whether the polyphenol content of olive oil matters for heart health.[62] Considering the wide variety of olive oils available now, this is an important question. Is it good enough to buy whatever's on sale, or is it worth seeking out a specialty store and spending a few extra dollars for high-polyphenol oil, which is typically more expensive?

Individuals consumed either low-, medium-, or high-polyphenol olive oils, and the results showed that the higher the polyphenol content, the higher the HDL and the lower their level of oxidized LDL. The authors wrote, "Olive oil is more than a monounsaturated fat. Its phenolic content can also provide benefits for plasma lipid levels and oxidative damage."[63] Hippocrates, a Greek physician often called "the father of medicine," said it best: "Let food be thy medicine and medicine be thy food."

How to Find Good Olive Oil[64]

Testing of olive oil reveals anywhere from 60 to 90 percent of the olive oils sold in American grocery stores and served in restaurants are adulterated with cheap, oxidized, omega-6 vegetable oils, such as sunflower oil or peanut oil, or non-human- grade olive oils, which are harmful to health in a number of ways. **Even "extra-virgin" olive oil is often diluted with other less expensive oils, including hazelnut, soybean, corn, sunflower, palm, sesame, grape seed and/or walnut. These added oils will not be**

listed on the label, so most people will not be able to discern that their olive oil is not 100 percent pure.

Similarly, the "use by" or "sell by" date on the bottle really does not mean a whole lot, as there's no regulation assuring that the oil will remain of high quality until that date. The date you really want to know is the "pressed on" date or "harvest" date, which are essentially the same thing because olives go bad almost immediately after being picked.

They're pressed into olive oil basically the same day they're harvested. High-quality olive oil is pressed within a couple of hours of picking. Poorer-quality olive oils may be pressed 10 hours after the olives are picked. Ideally the oil should be pressed in under an hour but certainly within a few hours. The harvest date should be less than six months old when you use it; but unfortunately, few olive oils actually provide a harvest date. As for olive oil in restaurants, more often than not, the olive oil served for bread dipping is typically of very poor quality and is best avoided.

Olive oil is extremely perishable even when used cold, thanks to its chlorophyll content, which accelerates decomposition. If you're like most people, you're probably leaving your bottle of olive oil right on the counter, opening and closing it multiple times a week. It's important to remember that any time the oil is exposed to air and/or light, it oxidizes, and the chlorophyll in extra-virgin olive oil accelerates the oxidation of the unsaturated fats. Clearly, consuming spoiled oil (of any kind) will likely do more harm than good. To protect your olive oil from rancidity, be sure to:

- Keep it in a cool, dark place
- Purchase smaller bottles to ensure freshness
- Immediately replace the cap after each pour

As for the best place to buy olive oil, look for stores where taste testing is allowed and encouraged, such as gourmet stores or specialty retailers.

So how can you distinguish superior olive oil from an inferior one, or tell whether your olive oil has gone bad? Here are four telltale signs to look out for:

1. **Rancidity.** If it smells like crayons or putty, tastes like rancid nuts and/or has a greasy mouthfeel, your oil is rancid and should not be used.

2. **Fusty flavor.** "Fusty" oil occurs when olives sit too long before they're milled, leading to fermentation in the absence of oxygen. Fusty flavors are incredibly common in olive oil, so many simply think it's normal. However, your olive oil should not have a fermented smell to it, reminiscent of sweaty socks or swampy vegetation. To help you discern this particular flavor, look through a batch of Kalamata olives and find one that is brown and mushy rather than purple or maroon-black and firm. The flavor of the brown, mushy one is the flavor of fusty.

3. **Moldy flavor.** If your olive oil tastes dusty or musty, it's probably because it was made from moldy olives, another occasional olive-oil defect.

4. **Wine or vinegar flavor.** If your olive oil tastes like it has undertones of wine and vinegar (or even nail polish), it's probably because the olives underwent fermentation with oxygen, leading to this sharp, undesirable flavor.

Here's a summary of various tips gathered from experts about how to find the best-quality olive oil:

- **Harvest date:** Try to purchase oils only from the current year's harvest. Look for "early harvest" or "fall harvest."

- **Storage and tasting:** Find a seller who stores the oil in clean, temperature-controlled stainless-steel containers topped with an inert gas such as nitrogen to keep oxygen at bay, and bottles it as they sell it; ask to taste it before buying.

- **Color and flavor:** According to Guy Campanile, an olive-oil producer, genuine, high-quality extra-virgin olive oil has an almost luminescent green color.

However, good oils come in all shades, from luminescent green to gold to pale straw, so color should not be a deal breaker.

The oil should smell and taste fresh and fruity, with other descriptors including grassy, apple, green banana, herbaceous, bitter, or spicy (spiciness is indicative of healthy antioxidants).

Avoid flavors such as moldy, cooked, greasy, meaty, and metallic, or resembling cardboard.

- **Bottles**: If buying prebottled oil, favor bottles or containers that protect against light; darkened glass, stainless steel, or even clear glass enclosed in cardboard are good options. Ideally, buy only what you can use up in six weeks.

- **Labeling terms**: Ensure that your oil is labeled "extra-virgin," since other categories—"pure" or "light" oil, "olive oil" and "olive pomace oil"—have undergone chemical processing.

  Some terms commonly used on olive-oil labels are meaningless, such as "first pressed" and "cold pressed."

  Since most extra-virgin olive oil is now made with centrifuges, it isn't "pressed" at all, and true extra-virgin oil comes exclusively from the first processing of the olive paste.

- **Quality seals**: Producer organizations such as the California Olive Oil Council and the Australian Olive Association require olive oil to meet quality standards that are stricter than the minimal USDA standards.

  Other seals may not offer such assurance. Of course, finding "USDA certified organic" is a bonus, but not the only consideration.

  Though not always a guarantee of quality, PDO (protected designation of origin) and PGI (protected geographical indication) status should inspire some confidence.

- **Storage and use**: Keep your olive oil in a cool and dark place, and replace the cap or cork immediately after each pour. Never let it sit exposed to air.

- **Prolonging freshness**: To slow oxidation, try adding one drop of astaxanthin to the bottle. Astaxanthin is red, so it will tint your olive oil.

  As the olive oil starts to pale, you know it's time to throw it away.

  Alternatively, add one drop of lutein, which is orange in color. Vitamin E oil is another option, but since it's colorless, it will not give you a visual indicator of freshness.

RIGHTING THE NUTRITIONAL SHIP

When it comes to dietary fats, we're in backwards world, where up is down, down is up, and the oils that have been promoted as being good for your heart health are just the opposite.

Excessive linoleic-acid consumption promotes oxidative stress (including oxidized LDL), chronic low-grade inflammation, hypertension, atherosclerosis, and heart arrhythmias. It is undoubtedly a major contributor to heart disease and overall cardiovascular disease, especially when consumed as industrial seed oils, and even more so when combined with a diet high in sugar and other refined carbohydrates. Whole foods high in LA do not seem to be as problematic, and in some instances they provide health benefits due to their inherent antioxidants, vitamins, minerals, healthy omega-3s, and other whole-food constituents that help protect the LA from oxidation. For example, most nuts and seeds are good sources of vitamin E, which is a potent antioxidant that may help protect the fragile omega-6 from being damaged.

However, in most industrialized nations, the majority of omega-6 no longer comes from whole foods, such as fish and other seafood, nuts, seeds, and eggs. It now comes from chemically unstable and easily damaged industrial seed oils. Since the average consumption of these industrial seed oils is around 40 to 55 grams per day in most of these societies, compared to an almost negligible EPA and DHA intake of just 0.1 to 0.3 grams per day, the omega-6-to-3 ratio has shifted from the one that kept us healthy and robust for millennia to one that promotes inflammation, atherosclerosis, and hypertension. **Reducing your intake of industrial seed oils and increasing marine and plant omega-3s may be one of the most *effective and simplest* strategies for reducing your risk for cardiovascular disease.**

Summary

- Many of the "facts" you've been told about the food you eat and how it relates to heart disease are wrong. Fats do not clog your arteries, salt does not cause hypertension, omega-3 fat does raise your cholesterol, but that's not necessarily a bad thing, because low cholesterol does not necessarily make you healthier.

- Omega-3s, specifically DHA and EPA, decrease platelet aggregation—blood clotting and small-dense LDL particles in the bloodstream.

- DHA and EPA are both proven to promote good health, but if you're working to promote *heart* health, DHA is more effective. This doesn't mean you should seek out only DHA, but look for supplements that contain higher levels of DHA than EPA.

- Olive oil, particularly high-quality extra virgin olive oil, contains oleic acid and polyphenol, which can dramatically reduce the susceptibility of LDL to oxidation and promote healthy lipid content.

CHAPTER 6

OMEGA-3 VERSUS OMEGA-6: FATS THAT *REGENERATE, NOT DEGENERATE*

As we've covered so far, nutrition and health experts have been advising you to make omega-6 fats a significant part of your diet in order to ensure a longer, healthier life, but this recommendation has resulted in a decline in overall health at a population level across multiple countries all over the world. On an individual level, it's likely made you sicker, heavier, and more inflamed. In this chapter, we'll look at brain development, as well as specific diseases and how they relate to the skewed omega-6-to-omega-3 ratio in the modern diet. Some illnesses may be exacerbated by an excess of adulterated omega-6 and a deficiency of omega-3, and some may be improved by setting this ratio right.

Recall from Chapter 3 that humans have the ability to convert the "parent" omega-6 and omega-3 fats into other fats in the same families. The conversion process requires multiple steps, each one controlled by an enzyme. Various health conditions affect the activity of these enzymes. Insulin resistance and type 2 diabetes are conditions whose incidence has skyrocketed in recent years, with over half of the U.S. having pre-diabetes or full-blown type 2 diabetes, and these conditions result in a reduction in the activity of one of the key conversion enzymes.[1,2]

On the other hand, insulin *increases* the actions of other enzymes involved in the conversion pathway. When the activity of the different enzymes is upregulated or downregulated— they're either working overtime or slacking on the job—the compounds produced along the way either accumulate or dwindle. Think of it like a factory assembly line: each worker along the length of the line has to be doing her job at the right pace or the entire production is compromised. It's the same way with converting the parent omega-6 and 3—linoleic acid and alpha-linolenic acid, respectively—into their downstream metabolites. In the case of ALA, those downstream metabolites are the critical factors that contribute to the synthesis of EPA and DHA, which are so lacking in our modern food supply.

Table 6.1 provides a look at why we need more long-chain omega-3 fats these days, owing to various natural processes, health conditions, and medications that interfere with the conversion process.

Table 6.1: Causes of Insufficient EPA and DHA and Why We Need More of These Fats

---

Excessive adulterated omega-6 linoleic acid in the diet (mainly from industrial seed oils such as soybean, cottonseed, corn, and safflower oils)

Inadequate ALA, EPA, and DHA in the diet

Chronic inflammatory states increase need for omega-3

- Air pollution and use of household cleaning and personal care products increase inflammation in the lungs and arteries
- Heavy metal accumulation

Reduced activity of conversion enzymes

Enzymes involved in the fatty-acid conversions require specific nutrients as essential cofactors. These include zinc, magnesium, biotin, and vitamin B6. Several factors interfere with absorption of these nutrients, potentially reducing the production of EPA and DHA:

- Medications
  - Antacids (including the commonly prescribed proton-pump inhibitors [PPIs], as well as other types of antacids)
  - Blood-pressure medications (ACE inhibitors, diuretics, calcium channel blockers)
  - Oral contraceptives
  - Statin drugs[3,4,5,6,7,8,9]
- Bariatric surgery
- Intestinal conditions that cause malabsorption of nutrients (Crohn's disease, ulcerative colitis, celiac disease, IBS, leaky gut)
- Agents that increase excretion of vitamins and minerals (caffeine, diuretics)

Insulin levels

- Chronically high insulin (those with type 2 diabetes or insulin resistance): high insulin = decreased ALA, insulin resistance = decreased EPA/DHA
- Low insulin levels (those with type 1 diabetes or advanced type 2 diabetes) = decreased EPA/DHA

Consumption of industrial trans fats

Hypothyroidism

Advanced age (conversion enzyme activity naturally decreases with age)

Menopause (lower estrogen levels may impair effective fat conversion)[10]

People with chronic low-grade inflammation can be thought of as being in a state of EPA and DHA deficiency. Aside from the health challenges the existing inflammation causes, the paucity of EPA and DHA can lead to additional problems, since there won't be enough EPA and DHA available to perform their normal, everyday roles in the body, such as serving as structural components in cell membranes. **Neurons in your brain are especially rich in DHA, so an inadequate DHA supply could potentially contribute to cognitive problems and unbalanced moods. When you look at the exploding incidence of dementia and depression in the Western world, you can't help but wonder if the dramatic decrease in omega-3 fats in our food supply is a major factor.**

Below is a list of diseases and other health complications associated with inadequate EPA and DHA—but keep in mind, this is just the short list, and it includes only the most common and most serious issues. Owing to the important roles these critical fats play in so much of human physiology, there are other, less severe problems that might also result from insufficient omega-3 over the long term.

Disease states associated with EPA/DHA deficiency:

- Insulin resistance
- Prediabetes
- Diabetes—especially diabetic retinopathy (eye damage) and neuropathy (nerve damage)
- Obesity
- Cardiovascular disease
- Hypertension
- Fatty liver or NASH (nonalcoholic steatohepatitis)
- Chronic kidney disease
- Peripheral vascular disease; peripheral arterial disease
- Coronary artery disease; coronary heart disease
- Ischemic stroke
- Airway inflammation (asthma, COPD)

- Acute respiratory distress syndrome
- Alzheimer's disease and other forms of dementia
- Age-related macular degeneration
- Depression
- Schizophrenia
- Anxiety
- Bipolar disorder
- Seasonal affective disorder
- Autoimmune diseases (including inflammatory bowel disease [Crohn's disease, ulcerative colitis], psoriasis, psoriatic arthritis, celiac disease, multiple sclerosis)
- Heart failure
- Periodontitis

ALA Conversion: It's Not a Given

Under ideal conditions, only a fraction of ALA is converted into EPA and DHA, and most people are operating under those ideal conditions, with optimum metabolic health or dietary choices. Some plant-based experts observe that those who are metabolically healthy and have enough ALA in their diet seem to have little problem in making this conversion, and effective conversion of ALA to DHA happens when the omega-6-to-3 ratio in the diet is about 3–4:1.[11] But people in most industrialized countries consume an omega-6-to-3 ratio of around 10:1, significantly reducing this conversion. So even though you can, technically, make this conversion, that doesn't mean it happens perfectly all the time.

Experienced bakers know that altitude, humidity, and other environmental factors affect the way a homemade cake turns out. It's the same with these fat conversions happening the right way: just because all the ingredients are assembled on the counter doesn't mean they'll spontaneously arrange themselves into a cake. They have to be blended together in just the right way, with each particular step happening at the right time. So it is with omega-3 fats in your body—it's not just a matter of having the raw materials on hand: conditions have to be right for them to produce the results you desire.

EARLY CHILDHOOD DEVELOPMENT: LONG-CHAIN OMEGA-3S ARE A BABY'S BRAIN'S BEST FRIEND

Omega-3 nutrition in early life—including in the womb—is a major factor in healthy brain development. And healthy brain development influences everything from cognition to attention span, the ability to focus, communicate, learn, and interact with the world. Considering the rising rates of attention deficit disorder (ADD), learning disabilities, and other issues that affect learning, cognitive function, and mood in children, it's possible that the average pregnant American woman's diet, so high in omega-6 and so low in omega-3, is contributing.

A high adulterated omega-6 intake, which we've established is bad news for your heart and overall health, may be especially undesirable during pregnancy because it reduces the amount of long-chain omega-3s available to the developing baby.[12] A high omega-6-to-3 ratio in pregnant mothers may lead to developmental problems in their babies, and supplementing premature infants with oils rich in DHA has been shown to reduce this risk.[13] Proper formation of the brain, and the healthy cognitive function this enables, doesn't only affect childhood. These nutritionally influenced processes at the very earliest stages of life have implications throughout adolescence and into adulthood,[14] so you want to do all you can to give your children the best possible start in life.

Women of childbearing age have the greatest capacity to convert ALA to EPA and DHA. This may be influenced by their higher estrogen levels, and it's likely yet another feature of human evolution and biology that persists with us to the current day: developing fetuses and newborn babies require a great deal of long-chain omega-3s, so mom better be getting plenty in her diet, or be able to make them from ALA, both during pregnancy and immediately after, to make sure there's enough in her breast milk after the baby is born. The average conversion rate of ALA to EPA and DHA in most people is about 0.2 to 8 percent and 0.05 percent, respectively, but it's as high as 21 percent and 9 percent, respectively, in young women.[15] However, considering how little ALA most people get, even young women with this relatively high conversion rate still end up with only a tiny amount of DHA. **Even if someone's rate of conversion is high, they can convert only what's available to *be* converted, and there typically isn't much ALA to begin with.**

The International Society for the Study of Fatty Acids and Lipids recommends that women who are pregnant or breastfeeding consume 300 mg per day of DHA. But the average pregnant or nursing woman's DHA intake is a paltry 60 to 80 mg a day—about 25 percent of the recommended amount.[16]

That women of childbearing age are so much better than men and older women at converting ALA to EPA and DHA suggests that these fats are particularly important to a growing fetus. DHA in particular is crucial for healthy development of the brain and the eyes, as it is the most prevalent polyunsaturated fatty acid in the central nervous system. The accumulation of DHA in babies occurs primarily during the third trimester[17] and continues into the first 6 to 10 months after birth.[18]

While a woman's overall diet can alter the fatty acid composition of her breast milk (the higher her omega-3 intake, the more omega-3 her milk will contain), on average the fats in breast milk are 0.5 to 1 percent ALA (omega-3), 0.4 to 0.7 percent arachidonic acid (an omega-6), 8 to 17 percent linoleic acid (LA), and just 0.3 to 0.6 percent DHA.[19] However, research suggests that for DHA levels in infants to reach their peak, breast milk should contain a bit more DHA—around 0.8 percent.[20]

Less than 1 percent of the fats in breast milk as DHA probably doesn't sound like much, but you'd be surprised just how critical even this small amount is. Remember, compared to saturated and monounsaturated fat in your diet, polyunsaturated fats in general make up only a small portion of total fat, but their impact is disproportionately high. It's just like vitamins and minerals: some of these nutrients are measured in milligrams or even *micrograms*—extraordinarily small amounts—but if you're deficient in something, it can have a massive effect on your health. It's especially important for moms to make sure they're getting enough EPA and DHA, because there's only one chance to ensure their babies get enough during their formative days and months. And women carrying twins need *even more* omega-3.[21]

Getting the balance of fats right isn't important only when a baby is in the womb. Babies' brains and nervous systems continue developing after they're born, and they need to have the right building blocks. The formation of neurons is complete before birth, but synthesis of several other types of cells is essential for proper brain function to continue after birth.[22] The formation of synapses—the spaces between neurons and the actual sites of cellular communication in the brain—depends on an adequate supply of DHA, as does synthesis of myelin, a fatty substance that surrounds and protects neurons like the rubber or plastic that insulates electrical cords on the appliances in your home.[23] It appears that babies will develop better cognitive performance when given DHA in their first few months.[24]

Neurons don't just orchestrate cellular communication in your brain. They also connect your brain to your muscles, which is what allows you to walk, run, throw a ball, blink, and even breathe. So the proper formation of neurons and the synapses between them—which is dependent on sufficient DHA[25]—is important for more than just your central nervous system. At the most basic level, this process is essential just to enable you to think and move.

DHA in early life is critical for healthy development throughout childhood and even into adulthood. Ensuring appropriate omega-3 supply during these important times not only helps with eye and brain development, but is also believed to impact cognition, learning, behavior, and even reproduction later in life.

Even though women of childbearing age are the rock stars of converting ALA to DHA, rock star is a relative term here: remember, the conversion is only about 9 percent, and most young women consume very little ALA to start with. Pregnant and breastfeeding mothers should aim for an omega-6-to-3 ratio of less than 4:1 in their diet, so they can be sure they're passing enough DHA on to their babies. According to one group of researchers, "All together, the evidence provided by studies in human infants indicate that despite the fact that the ALA-supplemented infant formula contributes efficiently to the maintenance of the omega-3 status in premature newborns, they have a modest impact on DHA levels and that these levels do not reach those observed in breastfed infants."[26] Just like adults, it seems babies are better off getting DHA directly, rather than relying on typically highly inefficient conversion from ALA.

Because DHA mostly accumulates during the third trimester, babies born prematurely miss out on their most important exposure to DHA. Breast milk contains DHA, so breastfed babies may be able to catch up—especially if mom's diet is high in DHA. Preemies who are breastfed have higher developmental scores at 18 months compared to those who are formula-fed, and preterm infants who are given breast milk for four weeks or longer have significantly higher IQ at seven to eight years of age compared to those who were fed exclusively with formula.[27] Breastfeeding also leads to better outcomes in cognitive development, vocabulary, visual-motor coordination, and behavior.[28,29,30] These are benefits that persist throughout childhood: breastfeeding, whether for preemies or full-term babies, is associated with better cognitive ability and educational achievement and fewer neurological abnormalities at nine years of age.[31,32] Want your babies to be intelligent and well adjusted? Make sure they have enough EPA and DHA.

Of course, it's not always possible for women to breastfeed. Be aware, though, that many commercial infant formulas provide only LA and ALA. This may be why babies fed formula lacking omega-3s have a higher incidence of learning disabilities later in life compared to breastfed babies.[33,34,35] Premature babies who are formula fed may be at especially high risk for DHA deficiency, and lack of this all-important fat is associated with numerous adverse outcomes, such as impaired cognition, poor eyesight, decreased learning ability, and altered behavior. That said, premature babies—and full-term babies—can still get a great start in life by consuming formulas fortified with omega-3s, especially in the form of EPA and DHA rather than ALA. **Whether babies are breastfed or formula-fed, the important thing is to ensure they have enough EPA and DHA.**

Recall from Chapter 5 that generous intake of omega-3s and cutting back on adulterated omega-6 helps keep blood pressure at a healthy level. Many pregnant women are at risk for pregnancy-induced hypertension and a related condition called preeclampsia. Higher amounts of long-chain omega-3s in their diet might reduce this risk. Inuit women living near the sea and consuming more omega-3s are almost three times less likely to develop hypertension in pregnancy compared to Inuit women living farther inland.[36,37] A lower maternal omega-3 index (the amount of omega-3 in red blood cells) is associated with greater risk of preeclampsia.[38] According to one study, a 15 percent increase in the ratio of omega-3 to omega-6 fats in red blood cells was associated with a 46 percent reduction in risk of preeclampsia, so even a modest change in the diet can yield a big benefit.[39]

To be fair, another study showed that pregnant women at high risk for developing hypertension had no significant benefit from supplementing with EPA/DHA.[40] The dose of omega-3 used in the study—2.7 grams—was pretty generous, but it's possible that the women had a typical high intake of omega-6, so even this amount of omega-3 may not have been enough to correct the imbalance. On balance, the bulk of the evidence indicates that DHA and EPA supplementation is beneficial for pregnant women and their babies.

DHA and EPA Recommendations for Pregnant Women and Breastfeeding Mothers

- Pregnant women should supplement with at least 300 mg of DHA per day. Greater amounts of marine omega-3s may be needed in women pregnant with twins or multiple babies and for women who have had multiple pregnancies, particularly if the pregnancies are close together (to ensure her omega-3 supply has been made replete since the previous pregnancy).

- Consuming high-quality fish oil or other marine oils like krill oil may be a safer strategy than consuming fish, as high-quality marine oils are in general processed to remove mercury and other harmful compounds.

- Breastfeeding mothers should supplement with DHA and EPA (especially DHA), particularly if their baby was born prematurely. We recommend at least 500 to 1,000 mg of EPA/DHA.

- Pregnant women and breastfeeding mothers should limit intake of adulterated omega-6 fats and industrial trans fats by reducing consumption of margarines, soybean-oil-based salad condiments, sandwich spreads, and processed foods containing soy, corn, cottonseed, and safflower oils.

- Formula-fed infants should get supplemental DHA or DHA and EPA if the formula does not contain adequate amounts of DHA (0.2% to 0.5% of total fat). You can add these fats to infant formula by poking a hole in a fish or krill oil capsule and squeezing the oil into the formula, or adding a very small amount from a bottle of liquid marine oil (fish oil or algal oil).

DEPRESSION AND MOOD DISORDERS

Considering the indispensable role of long-chain DHA and EPA in the brain, it stands to reason that insufficient EPA and DHA might be contributing to the epidemics of depression, anxiety, and other mood disturbances that afflict so many millions of people today. Of course, modern society changes more quickly than anyone can reasonably keep up with, and there's no shortage of non-dietary factors that could be contributing to this: financial worries, job stress, inadequate sleep, online bullying and aggression, pressure to have a certain physique, etc. But researchers believe that despite the relentless pace of life today, the progressive increase in depression in the industrialized world since World War II is unlikely to be entirely attributable to societal changes, changes in the criteria for diagnosis, or reporting bias.[41,42] In other words, it's not just that depression is being recognized more than it used to be, or simply that people who might not have been classified as having depression a few decades ago are falling into that category now. **Depression *is* increasing, not just our awareness of it.**

Depression itself is a difficult enough issue to contend with, but it's even more grim when you learn that as many as 30 to 40 percent of people with a major depressive disorder are considered "treatment-resistant," meaning their depression doesn't get any better with drugs or therapy.[43] **The rise in the incidence of depression has paralleled the rise in the consumption of vegetable oils. Major depressive disorder is estimated to become the second leading cause of disability worldwide by 2020, but populations that consume a lot of fish have a low prevalence of this illness.[44,45]**

However, back in Chapter 1, we learned from the mistakes of Ancel Keys and other researchers that we don't want to confuse correlation with causation. Just because people are consuming much less omega-3 and a lot more omega-6 than they used to, and there's a significant increase in depression and mood disorders than there used to be, doesn't automatically mean that the change in dietary fats is causing the unstable moods. But we're not playing the association game here. The science indicates that this dramatic shift in fats *is* at least partly responsible. Other things can and do contribute, of course, but when you have a more biologically appropriate balance of these fats in your diet *and in your brain*, those other things might be much easier to deal with.

In Chapter 4, we wrote about inflammation and how the modern diet makes some people's bodies act as if they're "on fire" from chronic, low-grade inflammation all the time. You probably tend to think of inflammation as it relates to physical pain, but inflammation can also occur in your brain, and the result may look and feel more like emotional and psychological pain, rather than a physical sensation. Excessive pro-inflammatory compounds and signaling molecules are found in patients with depression.[46] Healthy moods, a positive mental outlook, emotional resilience, and the ability to cope with everyday stressors depend on your brain generating and using the right balance of neurotransmitters—molecules like dopamine and serotonin, which you might know of as "feel-good chemicals." Researchers have noted that inflammatory compounds in your brain reduce the availability of the precursors and building blocks for these neurotransmitters and interfere with proper functioning of your hypothalamus and pituitary gland, which produce hormones that also contribute to balanced moods.[47,48] Some antidepressant medications appear to work in part by inhibiting release of these pro-inflammatory compounds.[49] But what if you ate a diet that resulted in less inflammation in the first place?

You may recall that omega-3 fats work by affecting some of the same biochemical pathways that aspirin does, and this partly explains their anti-inflammatory effects. *Partly* is the key word there, and here's the rest of the story: It used to be thought that omega-3s helped with inflammation by decreasing the production of inflammatory compounds. But more recent research has shown that in addition to this, EPA and DHA are precursors of compounds called *resolvins*, so named because they help resolve inflammation once it's already happened, as well as *protectins*, named for their role in protecting cells, particularly neurons in the brain, against damage and death.[50]

Joseph Hibbeln, M.D., a physician and U.S. Navy captain who conducts research at the National Institutes of Health, found that countries with populations that consume more fish have lower rates of depression.[51] Numerous studies confirm this finding,[52] showing populations that consume more fish having lower risks of suicidal ideation[53] and better mental-health status.[54] Patients with depression have lower levels of EPA and/or DHA in their blood or body fat.[55,56,57]

Returning to pregnant women for a moment, Hibbeln found an inverse correlation between postpartum depression and total seafood intake as well as DHA in mother's milk in 22 countries: the higher the seafood intake, and the higher the DHA in women's breast milk, the lower the incidence of postpartum depression.[58]

DHA and EPA may improve the effects of neurotransmitters in part by keeping cell membranes healthy. Remember, DHA is a primary constituent of neuronal membranes in the brain. The cell membrane is the outer perimeter, or boundary, of a cell; it's the point of contact between what's inside a cell and everything that's outside of it. If it's not built correctly—because it lacks adequate DHA and EPA—then things can't get into and out of the cell the way they're supposed to, including serotonin and dopamine.[59] Inadequate DHA and EPA in your brain may also affect the way your brain uses energy.[60] If you think about depression, it can be described as a kind of fatigue in your brain, or a low emotional energy state. A compound with a long name—phosphatidylserine—has been shown to have antidepressant effects, and long-chain omega-3s increase the amount of phosphatidylserine in brain-cell membranes.[61]

People living with depression often experience insomnia. It's not known for certain whether poor sleep contributes to depression or if depression makes it more difficult to sleep, but either way, the two are often intertwined. **Supplementation with 2 grams of EPA per day was shown to improve insomnia, depressed mood, and feelings of guilt and worthlessness when added to antidepressant therapy—a benefit that occurred within just three weeks.**[62] One study noted that, compared to placebo, 6.6 grams a day of EPA and DHA on top of standard antidepressant therapy in patients with major depressive disorder significantly improved scores on a commonly used depression assessment (the Hamilton Rating Scale for Depression) in just eight weeks.[63] If you or someone you know has ever experienced depression, especially if it was long-term, then you know how debilitating it can be, so a noticeable improvement in only three or even eight weeks is a ray of hopeful light in a very dark illness.

As we've said, compared to healthy individuals, people with depression typically have lower levels of EPA and DHA in their tissues.[64] Knowing now how important omega-3s are for brain health in general and for supporting balanced moods and proper neurotransmitter function in particular, it's not surprising that a meta-analysis of randomized controlled trials found that omega-3s are effective for improving major depressive disorder.[65] Most clinical trials testing marine omega-3s have found improvements in depressive disorders compared to placebo, and some have even found that DHA and EPA are equally effective as prescription antidepressants, such as fluoxetine (brand name Prozac).[66,67,68,69,70,71] As effective as prescription medication, with none of the side effects, and all those other benefits, too? Not too shabby for something that's been part of the human diet since the very beginning.

But as with cardiovascular disease, hypertension, and other conditions we've covered so far, increasing DHA and EPA aren't the only piece of this puzzle. It's also important to cut back on seed oils that are high in omega-6, which promote increased inflammation in your body and brain. A high intake of adulterated omega-6 is associated with increased risk of depressive and anxiety disorders, and we know that the effects of omega-3s are muted when in the context of a high omega-6 intake.[72,73,74] As with heart disease and overall health, so with depression and unstable moods: it's not enough just to tackle the problems on the back end by loading up on omega-3; you also want to stop the problems at their source by limiting the intake of adulterated omega-6.

BEHAVIORAL DISORDERS, MOOD DISTURBANCES, AND OTHER BRAIN DISORDERS

Depression is a leading cause of disability and reduced quality of life, but it's not the only unfortunate mental-health issue linked to insufficient omega-3 fats. When you think about the essential role of DHA and EPA in your brain, it's only logical that a host of other mood, behavioral, and psychological issues might result when there aren't enough of these fats to go around. And indeed, this is exactly what we see in things like ADHD, autism-spectrum disorders, bipolar disorder, and more. As is true for depression, there are likely multiple contributing factors generating these disorders, and these disorders have multiple subtypes. So a lack of DHA and EPA isn't the only thing driving them, but it's an important one, and it's one that is easily and inexpensively corrected.

ADHD, Autism Spectrum Disorders, and Dyspraxia

Attention Deficit Hyperactivity Disorder (ADHD) affects anywhere between 4 percent and 15 percent of school-aged children in the U.S.; and for many people, it continues into and throughout adulthood.[75] Children and adults with ADHD have lower levels of DHA and EPA, and this correlates with behavioral and learning problems, including poor conduct, hyperactivity and impulsivity, anxiety, tantrums, temper, and sleep difficulties.[76] A double-blind randomized controlled trial conducted in Japan showed that children with ADHD-like symptoms who were given omega-3 fortified foods (providing around 510 mg DHA and 100 mg EPA per day) were rated as having improved by their parents and teachers.[77] Another double-blind trial showed that compared to placebo, an omega-3 plus evening primrose-oil supplement significantly improved attention, behavior, and oppositional defiant disorder in children with ADHD-like symptoms.[78]

Children with autism-spectrum disorders (ASD) have also been found to have low DHA and total omega-3 fatty acid levels.[79] One report found DHA and EPA deficiencies in virtually 100 percent of ASD cases,[80] and 90 percent of patients with pervasive developmental disorder (PDD) have been found to have deficient DHA and EPA levels in their blood.[81] One double-blind trial in children aged 5 to 17 diagnosed with ASD found improvements in hyperactivity and stereotypy (persistent repetitive actions) when given 1.54 g a day of supplemental DHA and EPA.[82]

Dyspraxia, also known as developmental coordination disorder (DCD), is an impairment of gross and fine-motor function and coordination that affects approximately 5 percent of children.[83] ("Gross" and "fine" motor function encompass large and small movements, respectively, such as walking and jumping, but also handwriting and in some cases speech.) These children are also more likely to have learning, behavioral, and psychosocial issues as well. One double-blind trial found that in 117 children aged 5 to 12 with DCD, a supplement (80 percent fish oil, 20 percent evening primrose oil) providing a little over 700 mg of EPA and DHA with a much smaller amount of omega-6 (in a ratio of 4:1 omega-6-to-3) and vitamin E led to significant improvements in reading, spelling, and behavior over three months of treatment compared to an olive-oil placebo.

Mood and Aggression

One double-blind trial showed that DHA and EPA supplementation reduced anger, anxiety, and depressive states in healthy young adults after just 35 days.[84] The dose used was 1600 mg EPA and 800 mg DHA per day. Compare this to what the American Heart Association recommends for people without heart disease (two fatty-fish meals per week, which provides only around 500 mg of combined EPA and DHA) or those with heart disease (1,000 mg of long-chain omega-3s). Now, the subjects in the study were relatively healthy; it's possible that people with severe anxiety, depression, or other mood disorders, or with other physical health issues, would need even more.

Individuals with schizophrenia and borderline personality disorder may also benefit from supplemental omega-3s. Upon autopsy, schizophrenic patients have been found to have depleted levels of long-chain omega-3s.[85] As for borderline personality disorder, compared to placebo, 1 gram of EPA daily for eight weeks led to reductions in aggression and depressive symptoms in women with this illness.[86]

DHA and EPA may also reduce violence and suicides.[87,88] Lower levels of EPA have been noted in people who have attempted suicide.[89] In patients with recurrent self-harm, supplementing with about 2 grams of EPA and DHA daily led to improvements in depression, suicidality, and daily stresses.[90] Low levels of EPA and/or DHA have also been noted in social-anxiety disorder[91] and bipolar disorder.[92]

A review looking at pooled research on DHA and EPA supplementation concluded that "gold standard" double-blind, randomized, placebo-controlled trials consistently show combinations of DHA and EPA to benefit ADHD, autism, dyspraxia, dyslexia, and aggression. Research also supports a role for these long-chain omega-3s in improving bipolar disorder, with potential also for schizophrenia and borderline personality disorder, although more research is needed in these last two areas.[93]

Now, obviously, not everyone with low levels of DHA and EPA has poor mental health. But the correlation between low levels of long-chain omega-3s and a wide variety of mental health issues strongly indicates that there is a relationship between the two, combined with other factors.

Cognitive Decline and Alzheimer's Disease

As many as 40 percent of people over age of 85 may have dementia in some form.[94] This illness exacts a devastating emotional and financial toll on afflicted individuals and their loved ones and caregivers. The burden of illness from various forms of dementia and brain disorders may match or surpass that of cardiovascular disease and cancer.[95,96]

Patients with Alzheimer's disease have been found to have lower amounts of brain DHA compared to healthy individuals.[97] DHA and EPA are also important for insulin signaling in your brain and central nervous system, and brain insulin signaling may be disrupted in Alzheimer's disease. Recall our discussion of DHA and EPA for healthy brain development in babies? Your brain never stops developing. People of all ages need long-chain omega-3s, as they're especially important for memory, cognitive function, and brain plasticity.[98] With DHA playing such a crucial role in the physical structure of neurons, it's not an exaggeration to say *you cannot have healthy cognitive function without adequate DHA.*

People of all ages need DHA and EPA, but the elderly, particularly if they live on their own, may be less inclined than younger people to prepare a home-cooked meal that might naturally provide these fats. If they rely on packaged, processed foods for most of their meals, they're getting far more omega-6 than omega-3. Think about it: it's a lot easier for an 82-year-old man to prepare a microwave TV dinner than to grill a piece of salmon.

DHA is believed to make up 30 to 50 percent of all the fats in the mammalian brain.[99] Studies show that animals consuming diets high in omega-3 have increased concentrations of neurotransmitters, more receptors for these neurotransmitters (neurotransmitters don't do much good if they can't get into their target cells), increased neuron growth in the hippocampus (a brain region involved in memory and learning), higher concentrations of antioxidant enzymes, reduced concentrations of damaged brain-cell fats, better blood flow to your brain, and better memory.[100]

A high intake of fish is associated with a lower risk of dementia and Alzheimer's disease.[101,102] One study found that **individuals consuming fish once a week or more had a 60 percent lower risk of being diagnosed with Alzheimer's compared to those who rarely or never eat fish.**[103]

Alzheimer's and Insulin Resistance

Insulin resistance is a major risk factor for cognitive decline. Some researchers have even called Alzheimer's disease "insulin resistance of the brain" or "diabetes of the brain."[104] Alzheimer's disease and other forms of cognitive decline are also associated with a reduction in your brain's uptake and metabolism of glucose.[105] Glucose typically serves as your brain's primary fuel source, and PET scans show that Alzheimer's patients have substantial reductions in brain-glucose uptake (up to 20 percent in some areas).[106] What this means is that some forms of dementia may simply be a result of the brain "starving" for energy.

However, glucose isn't the *only* fuel your brain can use. Ketones are another molecule your brain can use for energy. If you're mindful of current understanding on health and nutrition, you've no doubt heard of ketogenic diets. (In fact, Dr. Mercola has written a best-selling book, *Fat for Fuel,* about how to optimize cyclical ketogenesis.) The intention of this approach is to improve mitochondrial function by helping your body regain the metabolic flexibility to burn fat as a primary fuel and allow your body to produce water-soluble fats called ketones.

Since ketones can serve as an important energy source for your brain, a number of studies have shown them to be useful for people with Alzheimer's and other forms of cognitive impairment. The best fats to help your body generate ketones are medium-chain triglycerides and, even better, caprylic acid, which has only eight carbons and is relatively easily metabolized to ketones.

Insulin resistance, which plays such an important part in Alzheimer's, impairs your body's ability to produce ketones. Ketones are generally produced only when carbohydrate availability and insulin levels in your body are low. As a hormone, insulin has multiple functions, one of which is to signal your body that you've just eaten. If you consume a typical Western diet, with many carbohydrates, your insulin level typically rises after a meal, letting your body know there's plenty of glucose (from carbs) to go around, so you don't *need* to make ketones for energy.

If you have insulin resistance, your brain faces a double whammy in terms of starving for energy: glucose is not being used efficiently, and high insulin levels prevent appreciable generation of ketones, so your brain doesn't get enough of *either* fuel. Insulin resistance undoubtedly leads to a reduction in the fuel supply available to your brain, and it's a major risk factor for cognitive problems. But remember what you learned about insulin resistance in Chapter 4: it's not solely about carbs. Your brain needs adequate DHA in order to be able to take up glucose properly. And since EPA increases fat burning, which could lead to higher ketone production, supplementation with both EPA and DHA may help to supply an aging, insulin-resistant brain with these nourishing ketones *and* potentially make it easier for your brain to use glucose as well.[107]

Postmortem studies have confirmed that Alzheimer's patients, as well as those with cognitive impairment but not dementia, have reduced brain and blood DHA levels compared to healthy people.[108,109,110,111,112] Higher intake of DHA and EPA is associated with a decreased risk of cognitive decline, so getting plenty of this fat in your diet might be a good tool in your arsenal to potentially prevent cognitive impairment.[113] Animal studies have shown that deficiency of long-chain DHA and EPA can reduce brain-glucose uptake by as much as 30 to 40 percent.[114] It's not that the glucose isn't *there;* it's that the brain isn't taking it in. Having enough DHA helps the brain accept that glucose.

Ten to 15 percent of patients with mild cognitive impairment will develop full-blown dementia within a year of being diagnosed, and these individuals have been found to have low blood levels of EPA and DHA.[115] In the Framingham Heart Study, which followed 899 men and women free of dementia for over nine years, **subjects whose DHA levels were the highest had a nearly 40 percent lower risk of developing dementia compared to subjects with the lowest levels.**[116]

In a double-blind randomized controlled trial, patients with a very mild degree of cognitive dysfunction had a slower cognitive decline compared to subjects on the placebo when supplemented with DHA (1.7 grams/day) and EPA (0.6 grams/day) for six months. When those who started off in the placebo group were switched over to the omega-3 supplement, they also showed a slowing in cognitive decline, but unfortunately, those with more advanced cognitive decline and Alzheimer's disease did not show benefit from the omega-3s, so it may be that there's a window of opportunity during which cognitive function and neuronal health are intact enough that they can be impacted positively by a greater supply of DHA and EPA. There may be a threshold or a "point of no return" after which damage is too severe and long-standing for the fats to make much difference.[117] Bottom line? **Start supplementing with marine omega-3s earlier rather than later to protect cognitive function.**

DHA and EPA are important for reducing your risk of and treating both dementia and cognitive impairment without dementia. A meta-analysis of double-blind placebo-controlled trials found that in those with cognitive impairment but without dementia, DHA and EPA supplementation led to improvements in immediate recall, attention, and processing speed. No benefit was found in those who had Alzheimer's disease, which again suggests that there might be a threshold after which interventions that are promising in those with milder impairment are no longer effective.[118]

In one study of 39 Alzheimer's patients, compared to placebo, and compared to omega-3s alone, a combination of DHA and EPA and alpha-lipoic acid resulted in a slower decline in overall cognition and performance of activities of daily living, as measured by a commonly used assessment tool, the Mini-Mental State Examination (MMSE). Considering the role of insulin resistance and impaired glucose metabolism in your brain as major factors in Alzheimer's disease, it makes sense that DHA and EPA together with ALA showed benefit compared to the placebo, and even compared to omega-3s on their own. By targeting the glucose and insulin problem as well as the fatty-acid status that may be contributing to impaired cognition, this combination is a one-two punch striking Alzheimer's at the cellular energy level.[119]

To the extent that Alzheimer's disease really is "brain insulin resistance" or "diabetes of the brain," then it's not too far off from type 2 diabetes in that protecting yourself against this dreaded illness—to the extent that any of us *can* protect ourselves—starts with getting the refined carbs out of your diet. But equally important is getting the bad *fats* out of your diet and getting the good ones in.

Below is a summary of the effects fats can have on your brain health.

Negative effects of DHA and EPA deficiency in your brain:[120]

- Impaired cell membrane function
- Decreased energy generation in neurons
- Increased levels of inflammatory compounds
- Decreased phosphatidylserine content
- Decreased dopamine levels and dopamine receptor activity
- Decreased blood flow to your brain
- Reduced availability of growth factors to support healthy neurons

- Decreased amino-acid delivery across your blood-brain barrier (amino acids are the building blocks for serotonin, dopamine, and other neurotransmitters)

Conditions that may benefit from DHA and EPA:

- Alzheimer's disease[121,122]
- Attention deficit hyperactivity disorder (ADHD)[123]
- Autism[124]
- Depression[125,126]
- Borderline personality disorder (mood instability and impulsive aggression)[127]
- Schizophrenia[128]
- Hostility[129]
- Anxiety[130]
- Bipolar disorder[131,132]
- Seasonal affective disorder[133]

OXIDATION OF OMEGA-6 FAT DRIVES NEURODEGENERATION

We've spent a fair amount of time focusing on the importance of omega-3 fats and what can happen if you don't have enough of them in your diet. Now let's dig a little deeper into the detrimental effects of excessive omega-6. Remember, vegetable oils, which are the predominant sources of omega-6 in the Western diet, are the fats government, medical, and nutrition authorities specifically advised you to consume after they erroneously determined saturated fats were to blame for every health problem under the sun. So if you've been trying to do the right thing by following this advice, let's definitively set the record straight.

As we've discussed, fatty acids—all kinds, including saturated, monounsaturated, and polyunsaturated—are primary elements in all your cell membranes. Your cell membranes are like security guards defending the perimeter of each and every cell: they let in good things like vitamins and minerals, and keep out bad things like toxins and waste products. If your cell membranes are going to do their job correctly, they must be built correctly, which means they have to have a healthy makeup of fats, and these fats have to be intact and undamaged. You wouldn't try to build a log cabin with rotting wood.

There are a wide variety of factors that contribute to oxidation, or damage, of these fragile fats: microorganisms (bacteria and other infectious agents), air pollution, smoking, poor diet, and other insults can damage the fats in your cell membranes. Recall from earlier that the chemical structure of a fat determines how susceptible it is to oxidation. The more double bonds a fat has, the more easily it's oxidized. This is why saturated fats, which have no double bonds, are the most stable, and polyunsaturated fats, which have two or more double bonds, are the most easily damaged. This oxidation of structural fats is thought to contribute to Parkinson's disease, Alzheimer's disease, schizophrenia, atherosclerosis, inflammation, and much more. These oxidized fats can wreak havoc with your health if they get incorporated into your cell membranes.[134]

If this seems like the kind of stuff that put you to sleep in high school biology or college biochem class, perk up, because this is vital to understand. If your cell membranes aren't built properly, then biological molecules that are designed to be embedded in or anchored to these membranes aren't going to work properly, either.

What are these biological molecules? For starters, there are insulin receptors, glucose transporters, thyroid hormone receptors, LDL receptors, and receptors and transporters for all kinds of hormones, enzymes, nutrients, and other compounds that, taken as a whole, *keep you alive and functioning well.*

Don't underestimate the importance of something as seemingly mundane and meaningless as your cell membranes. When you realize that just about everything that happens inside you occurs because each individual cell—be it a liver cell, a muscle cell, a neuron, a pancreatic cell—does what it's designed to do, you gain an appreciation for what an amazing orchestra your body is, with each one of your *trillions* of cells playing its part but also blending in seamlessly with all the others. Your membranes are anything *but* mundane and meaningless. Health begins at the cellular level, and if your cell membranes aren't healthy, then quite simply *you* won't be healthy.

When fats are oxidized in your cells, it can set off a chain reaction that causes other biological molecules to become damaged as well, including DNA and proteins.[135] Alzheimer's disease, Parkinson's disease, and other neurological and neurodegenerative disorders have among their hallmarks the buildup of abnormal and malfunctioning proteins. These dysfunctional proteins might not be the primary causes of these conditions, but as they accumulate and reach toxic levels inside and outside cells, they certainly worsen the process.

Adding insult to cellular injury, the destructive chain reaction of oxidation and damage doesn't stay localized to just one cell. Oh no, that would be too easy. Most cells are close enough to each other that the molecules that cause oxidation—free radicals—can jump from one cell to another, and another, on and on, spreading like dominoes until they reach an area that has enough *antioxidants* to neutralize them."[136]

Since cell membranes—especially the ones in your brain and central nervous system—are so rich with polyunsaturated fats, your body seems to interpret the oxidation of these fats as a signal that damage is occurring, and to mount a response to repair the cellular damage.[137] Damaged fats are like the alarm going off at a fire station, telling the firefighters to put on their gear and run to the truck.

DHA seems to be the canary in the coal mine in terms of sounding the oxidation alarm. DHA has *six* double bonds, so it's extremely fragile and highly susceptible to oxidation. (DHA stands for docosa*hex*aenoic acid, with "hex" meaning six, like a hexagon.) If a cell has been so highly damaged that it's safer for it to sacrifice itself rather than "infect" nearby cells, it commits cellular suicide, a process called *apoptosis*. But if a cell membrane doesn't have enough DHA in it, the warning bells might never go off, leaving this damaged cell to replicate and spread. Damaged cells replicating and spreading . . . if that sounds like cancer, now you understand how important adequate DHA is to health, from the very smallest part of you on up to your life as a whole.

MITOCHONDRIAL DYSFUNCTION

If you follow health and nutrition news, or if you read Dr. Mercola's book *Fat for Fuel*, you're probably familiar with mitochondrial dysfunction. It is important because some of the conditions we talked about earlier—especially depression and Alzheimer's disease—may be due in part to an energy shortage in certain areas of your brain. And where is energy generated? In your mitochondria!

Your mitochondria (singular *mitochondrion*) are responsible for producing most of your body's ATP (adenosine triphosphate), or the energy currency of your body. A couple of cell types, such as red blood cells and skin cells, don't have mitochondria, but just about every other cell does. In fact, some cells actually have *thousands* of mitochondria. And if your mitochondria become damaged, then your cells won't have enough energy, which directly contributes to virtually every chronic disease we know of. Most neurodegenerative disorders are associated with mitochondrial dysfunction in neurons. Besides Alzheimer's, this applies to Parkinson's disease, multiple sclerosis, and ALS (amyotrophic lateral sclerosis, a.k.a. Lou Gehrig's disease), just to name a few.

So what *causes* mitochondrial dysfunction? The primary thing is the oxidative damage from consuming too many carbs and omega-6, which reduces your ability to burn fat as your primary fuel. But for now, we are going to focus on the damage to fats in your tissues. Just like your cells themselves, all the mitochondria in your cells are surrounded by their own membrane. In fact, your mitochondria have *two* membranes, one on the outside and one forming an inner compartment. And just like your cell membranes, your mitochondrial membranes are composed mostly of fats. If these membranes are built with the wrong fats or become damaged, then your mitochondria become dysfunctional. Oxidized omega-6 linoleic acid and its byproducts have been specifically shown to damage mitochondria and impair healthy cellular function.[138,139]

Things generally go one of two ways with mitochondrial dysfunction. When your cells have insufficient energy and they're "starved" for long enough, they may deteriorate and eventually die, as happens in Alzheimer's, Parkinson's, and ALS. On the other hand, they might *refuse* to die. We mentioned the process of apoptosis—programmed cell suicide. Your mitochondria control this process, so if they're malfunctioning, they may not be able to properly engage the "kill switch," which could result in these damaged cells continuing to replicate unabated and eventually spreading to other parts of your body, wreaking havoc on the whole neighborhood.

ALLERGIES AND ASTHMA

If you feel like people seem to have more allergies these days than they used to, you're not wrong. If you have a school-aged child, it's hard to ignore how many children and young adults nowadays have life-threatening allergies to certain foods. Allergies are certainly nothing new, but they sure seem to affect more people than ever before.

The prevalence of allergies and allergic diseases in the industrialized world has increased so dramatically that it's not reasonable to attribute it to genetics, and the fact that so many children have severe allergies and allergic diseases tells us this isn't a matter of "just getting older." Something else is driving this increase. Our physical environment has changed, of course. There's more air pollution, pesticides, toxic ingredients in personal care products and cleaning agents, and any one of these, let alone all of them combined, could be causing people's immune systems to be on high alert. But it's also possible the Western diet has something to do with it.

The astonishing increase in the omega-6-to-3 ratio during the past hundred-plus years has paralleled the rise in the prevalence of allergic diseases such as rhino-conjunctivitis (nasal congestion, runny nose, sneezing, postnasal drip, red eyes, itchy nose or eyes), allergic asthma, and atopic eczema.[140] Many of the inflammatory compounds formed from omega-6 fats have been implicated in allergic asthma and other allergic diseases. A high omega-6 diet keeps susceptible individuals in a "hyperallergic" state, as opposed to omega-3s, which calm things down.

Remember, omega-6s and omega-3s compete for the same biochemical pathways—pathways that generate inflammatory and pro-allergenic compounds, or pathways that generate anti-inflammatory and anti-allergenic compounds. The more omega-6 you consume, the more the balance is tipped toward the inflamed, hypervigilant immune state. The combination of cutting back on adulterated omega-6 and increasing omega-3, encouraging formation of resolvins (those compounds formed from omega-3s that "resolve" inflammation), may help to reduce chronic inflammation and the chronic allergic state.

A systematic review and meta-analysis of 15 studies determined that pregnant women may be able to reduce their children's risk for allergic diseases by consuming adequate EPA and DHA.[141] The vast majority of the data show a reduced incidence of allergic diseases in children whose mothers had a higher intake of long-chain omega-3s during pregnancy. Reductions were confirmed for eczema and allergy to egg, and there were also reductions in sensitivity to any food and to any positive skin-prick test (wherein they test for multiple allergens) for at least the first year of life.[142]

Compared with consistent high fish intake during pregnancy, not eating fish at all is associated with a 30 percent increased risk of asthma in offspring by age five. It's also correlated with a 46 percent increased risk of a child being hospitalized for asthma and a 37 percent increased risk for being prescribed medication for asthma by age five.[143] A higher maternal dietary omega-6-to-3 ratio in pregnancy is associated with a 37 percent greater risk for allergic rhinitis in children by five years of age,[144] and consuming about 7 ounces or more of fish per week during pregnancy is associated with a 43 percent reduction in the risk of eczema in offspring.[145] Compared to never eating fish, eating fish even just once a week during pregnancy was shown to correlate with a 43 percent reduction in eczema and a 72 percent in hay fever in children at five years old.[146] It's true that "you are what you eat," but it's also true that you are what your *mother* ate, or if you're a pregnant woman or a woman looking to conceive, your children will be what *you* eat.

CANCER

We've mentioned briefly how oxidized and damaged fats in cell and mitochondrial membranes could facilitate a cell's transition from being healthy to turning cancerous. This alone tells you that you want to maintain an optimal omega-6-to-3 ratio, but there's more to this story. Anti-inflammatory metabolites from DHA and EPA may help to reduce the growth and invasiveness of tumors,[147,148,149] while linoleic acid (LA) can actually reverse the antiproliferative effects of EPA (inhibition of cancer growth), thereby increasing tumor growth.[150] LA has been shown to increase signaling compounds that promote angiogenesis (making new blood vessels to supply cancer cells and tumors) and increase the ability of cancer cells to invade other tissues and metastasize or spread to other parts of the body, while EPA and DHA help to inhibit this.[151]

For people already living with cancer, EPA and DHA may be a helpful adjunct to their treatment. One group of researchers found that EPA and DHA supplementation during chemotherapy or radiation helped to prolong survival without negatively impacting the effects of the conventional therapies.[152]

Having sufficient DHA and EPA may also boost the efficacy of cancer drugs. For these drugs to work, they have to get into the cancerous cells, and cell membranes that have adequate EPA and DHA are more permeable to these drugs, meaning the drugs get inside the cells more easily. Cancer agents that pass through the cell membrane directly (rather than through a special tube or channel within the membrane) are taken into cancer cells more readily when the membranes contain more of these unsaturated fats.[153] In fact, some cancer cells that develop a resistance to chemotherapy drugs may pull off this terrible stunt by reducing their membrane fluidity, making it more difficult for the drugs to get inside. According to one researcher, "Dietary supplementation with certain fats, including EPA, DHA, and GLA . . . may provide a means of enhancing the response to cancer therapies. Altering the physical and functional properties of tumor cell membranes by enrichment with these fats may increase the response to chemotherapy and radiation, and may, to some degree, reverse the resistance of cancer cells to certain chemotherapeutic agents."[154]

Please note that we're not saying all cancer is caused by inadequate omega-3 and too much omega-6 (although it's certainly possible that some cancers are). Cancer is a highly complex, multifactorial illness with numerous contributing factors, many of which researchers probably haven't even identified yet. We're simply showing you that increasing omega-3 and decreasing omega-6 in your diet might give you an edge when it comes to fighting this dreaded disease. With cancer, even a slight edge is surely better than nothing.

How's that for a whirlwind tour of the surprising effects of omega-6 and omega-3 fats on health? When you do something as frequently as eating—three times a day every day for most people—it's easy to take the implications for granted. But it's precisely *because* you do it so frequently that its implications are so profound. As we've discussed, getting your fats right—more good fats, fewer bad fats—can help you stay healthy, physically and mentally, body and mind, from the cradle to the grave.

In the next chapter, we'll shift focus from the exploding burden of chronic disease to another issue, the increased incidence of which has also paralleled the change in our dietary fats: obesity.

Summary

- Inadequate omega-3 intake can have a profound and negative impact on your mental and physical health.

- Beginning in utero and into early childhood, brain development in infants requires a nutritional intake high in DHA specifically, either through breastfeeding or through supplemented formula.

- Depression, mood disorders, and various mental-health disorders can be caused or worsened by low levels of long-chain omega-3s, and can be improved or alleviated with sufficient supplements of DHA and EPA.

- Cognitive decline, including Alzheimer's disease, is strongly attributed to omega-3 deficiency, and if remedied early enough, the effects can be offset.

- Oxidized fats, frequently from industrial seed oils, cause cell membranes to malfunction, inhibiting nearly all bodily functions. When these fats oxidize in the membranes of mitochondria, the cell's power plant, energy depletion contributes to degenerative mental diseases.

- Asthma and allergies are essentially forms of inflammation, and like inflammation, they can be controlled with adequate intake of DHA and EPA.

- Oxidized fats on cell and mitochondrial membranes can cause a cell to transition from healthy to cancerous, and EPA and DHA supplements can help slow this transition, enhancing response to cancer therapies.

CHAPTER 7

FATS THAT MAKE YOU LEAN, FATS THAT MAKE YOU FAT

The consumption of a Western diet—one composed primarily of processed food—has over the last century resulted in an epidemic of obesity with over two-thirds of Americans being overweight or obese.[1] But what you might *not* know is that **you can look thin on the outside, yet still be fat.** *Huh?* It's true!

This is a condition where you have an unhealthy amount of body fat, but instead of the so-called "subcutaneous" fat—which is just underneath the skin and is the fat you love to hate on your upper arms, thighs, or backside—the fat is deposited in areas where it shouldn't be, and where you can't see it, such as in and around your liver and pancreas.[2]

This hidden fat is called "visceral" fat, because it surrounds your internal organs (a.k.a. the *viscera*), and this kind of fat is far more harmful than the jiggly fat on your arms or hips.[3] People casually call this TOFI—thin outside, fat *inside*, and in the scientific research world, it is termed "normal weight obesity," which hints at exactly what it is: you can be at a normal weight, yet have abnormal blood work and the kinds of metabolic problems doctors would expect in an obese person.

Worldwide, the median prevalence of fatty-liver disease is 20 percent.[4] However, between 33 percent and 46 percent of American adults have fatty-liver disease, which interferes with the many critical functions the liver performs, especially blood sugar regulation.[5,6] With this in mind, it shouldn't surprise you that 52 percent of adults in the U.S. are diabetic or prediabetic,[7] since fat building up in the liver is a major contributor to type 2 diabetes. If this issue isn't resolved soon, the economic burden of these health issues will likely bankrupt the nation quicker than you can say "French fries."

Certain fats are more likely than others to result in storing harmful visceral fat. But the problem isn't just the storage of this fat; it's when stored fat shifts from an anti-inflammatory state to a pro-inflammatory state. Stored body fat isn't inert. It doesn't just sit there quietly like an innocent bystander while the rest of your body goes about its business. Think of stored fat as an endocrine gland that sends signaling molecules to the rest of your body—or better yet, think of it like a radio station: stored fat "broadcasts" messages that are received by other parts of the body, which do what the messages tell them to do. For example, this stored fat might tell your blood vessels to constrict, leading to elevated blood pressure.

The change in fat from an anti-inflammatory state to a pro-inflammatory state results in chronic, low-grade systemic inflammation, and the cellular messengers (called *cytokines*) that are released by inflamed fat cells influence a host of disease states that reads like a who's who of the chronic conditions that plague millions of Americans: insulin resistance, type 2 diabetes, high blood pressure, and cardiovascular disease. And those are just the biggies. Inflammatory cytokines also contribute to issues that are less devastating but still unpleasant, such as acne, dry skin, and menstrual cramps. A good marker of inflammatory fat is the amount of fat stored in your liver, which is increased by three main dietary factors:

1. **Refined sugar:** mostly in the form of added sugars, like sucrose ("table sugar") and high-fructose corn syrup, but also sugars you might consider "natural," such as 100 percent fruit juice

2. **Industrial seed oils:** cottonseed, safflower, soybean, corn, and sunflower oils

3. **Low intake of omega-3 fats:** particularly EPA and DHA

Of those three factors, consuming industrial seed oils is likely the worst offender for shifting body fat from being anti-inflammatory to pro-inflammatory, but as always it's compounded by a low intake of omega-3 fats, particularly EPA and DHA but also ALA. When your body is in a chronic state of low-grade inflammation, it's like a barbecue grill where the coals are still hot and smoldering and occasional embers get tossed around. If you consume excess omega-6 seed oils on top of this, it's like someone coming along and pouring gasoline on the red-hot coals: with fuel added to the fire, it'll rage out of control. In order to repair the situation, you need to change your dietary-fat intake so you can start to cool the fire within.

As we explained in Chapter 4, a small amount of acute, controlled inflammation is healthy and actually necessary for optimum biological function. It's only long-term, chronic, unresolved inflammation that you need to worry about, and while many things contribute to this kind of inflammation, a high intake of omega-6 fat paired with too little omega-3 ranks near the top of the list.

How can you *tell* if you have harmful hidden inflammatory fat? Work with your doctor to identify signs of fatty-liver disease, as liver fat is a good measure of whether you have hidden inflammatory fat elsewhere in your body. Later, we'll discuss strategies to reduce your risk of accumulating inflammatory fat and help you decrease inflammatory fat if you already have it.

Here's a summary of healthy versus harmful fat.[8]

Harmful Fat:

- **Ectopic fat with local effects:** fat in and around the kidneys and heart muscle, which mostly affects these areas

- **Ectopic fat with systemic effects:** fat in and around the liver, pancreas, and skeletal muscles, which affects your whole body

Healthy Fat:

- **Subcutaneous fat:** the fat just below your skin; the visible fat you typically think of as body fat

OMEGA-3-DEFICIENT FAT IS INFLAMED FAT

Inflamed visceral and subcutaneous fat have a deficit of the resolvins and protectins that help neutralize and protect against inflammation. Patients with peripheral vascular disease have markedly inflamed fat with a shortage of these DHA-derived compounds.[9,10] One study found that metabolites from DHA "are potent pro-resolving mediators that counteract both local cytokine production."[11] When your stored body fat is deficient in omega-3s, there's nothing to put the brakes on the inflammatory signals it sends out. On the other hand, if your fat tissue had enough omega-3s, it might be able to keep its own inflammatory state in check.

Fat tissue that's low in omega-3s is made even more inflammatory because the enzyme that inactivates these specialized inflammation-cooling compounds is unregulated in fat tissue.[12] This means there's more inflammation, combined with a lower capacity to control it. It's almost as if someone started a fire, and firefighters are on their way to the scene, but as the fire grows and spreads, the firefighters somehow get word that they're not needed, so they return to the firehouse. The inflammation is still there, and getting worse, but now your body is blocked from doing anything about it.

Restoring omega-3s in obese animals has been shown to reverse the deficiency of omega-3 pro-resolving compounds and shift the fat tissue to an anti-inflammatory state.[13] Giving resolvins or protectin-precursors from DHA to obese and diabetic mice improves insulin resistance in fat tissue, reduces the expression of inflammatory cell signals, and improves glucose tolerance while also lowering fasting glucose levels—all of which improve overall metabolic health.[14,15] Results from studies in mice and other animals don't automatically translate to humans, but they do provide useful information that we can formulate ideas from, so they're worth paying attention to.

Bottom line: compounds that are made from DHA help to reduce inflammation through multiple pathways. And when inflammation is reduced in this way—at the cellular level, by changing the types of molecules different tissues secrete—your body's overall state of inflammation is reduced, which means reduced risk for developing a debilitating condition driven by chronic systemic inflammation, or improvement of symptoms if you're already living with one or more of these.

Researchers have said that boosting the production of anti-inflammatory compounds from omega-3 fats is an important part of a strategy to combat inflammation in fat tissue.[16] An adequate supply of DHA and EPA ensures that your body has a pool of raw material from which to create these compounds. These anti-inflammatory compounds are so powerful that you shouldn't be surprised if pharmaceutical companies eventually develop medications derived from them that can be delivered via injection directly into visceral fat stores. If they ever do, though, no doubt they'll cost a fortune, so your best bet is simply to cut back on vegetable oils and eat more clean seafood or take high-quality fish- or krill-oil supplements.

OMEGA-6 DRIVES OBESITY AND INFLAMED FAT

Did you know that each of your fat cells can expand nearly 1,000-fold in volume and 10-fold in diameter?[17] They're like balloons that can fill, fill, and fill some more without popping. Only instead of being filled with helium, your fat cells are filled with, well, fat, of course.

The expansion of your fat cells is driven in part by chronic low-grade inflammation, which can be assessed by the presence of inflammatory compounds in your blood. These inflammatory compounds are like messages that tell your fat cells to suck up fat and hold onto it. And think about this for a second: we haven't said anything about calories or carbs here. They aren't really the problem. The dysregulation in your fat cells, which makes them hoard fat and hold on tight, is driven mostly by the *kind* of fat you eat, the kind of fat that gets incorporated into your fat cells, and the kinds of signals it sends out.

Where do these inflammatory compounds come from? One of the main sources is the omega-6 linoleic acid (LA) in your fat stores. As you know, out of all the different types of fats stored in your fat cells, LA is the most prevalent, and it is susceptible to conversion to pro-inflammatory mediators called *oxidized LA metabolites* (OXLAMs). The massive increase in LA in the Western diet—and in people's body fat—has paralleled the rise in chronic disease in the U.S., including obesity and type 2 diabetes.[18] Not surprising, considering what you now know about LA *encouraging* the storage of fat.

But all hope is not lost! Supplementation with a special type of fat, called *gamma-linolenic acid* (GLA), from borage oil, has been shown to reduce some of these fat-storing signals in as little as two weeks.[19] Other ways to decrease these signals include consuming more EPA and DHA, and more oleic acid (found in olive oil, avocados, and macadamia nuts),[20] as well as cutting back on LA. Avoiding processed foods full of corn, soybean, and cottonseed oils is a small price to pay for eating delicious foods that are high in *healthy* fats—and maybe even losing weight in the process!

In case you're feeling a little overwhelmed at this point, here are some simple ways to reduce inflammatory body fat:

- Reduce intake of industrial seed oils (cottonseed, soybean, corn, safflower, sunflower)

- Increase intake of GLA (borage oil, evening primrose oil, or black currant seed oil)

- Increase intake of oleic acid (olive oil, avocado, macadamia nuts)

- Increase intake of healthy omega-3 fats (ALA, EPA, DHA)

Concerned about Weight Loss?

If improving your omega-6-to-omega-3 ratio can help improve some of the adverse effects of inflammation and insulin resistance, it's possible that maintaining a proper ratio might even serve to outright prevent some of the illnesses that stem from these issues. As the saying goes, an ounce of prevention is worth a pound of cure, so don't wait until you're already sick to start paying attention to how much omega-6 and omega-3 you're eating. Getting the right balance of these fats in your diet should become a daily habit, like brushing your teeth. It may take some effort at first, but after a while, it'll be second nature and you won't even have to think about it.

What about alpha-linolenic acid (ALA)? We've emphasized EPA and DHA because these long-chain marine fats are the most potent of the omega-3s and they perform various functions ALA simply isn't capable of. But that doesn't mean the plant-sourced parent omega-3 is not biologically useful. Far from it. Research suggests ALA helps stimulate the burning of fat for fuel in muscle cells as well as in fat cells themselves.[21]

If you've struggled to lose weight, don't underestimate the importance of getting the right kinds of fat in your diet. This is especially important if you have a hard time kicking a sweet tooth. In a study of mice fed a diet high in fat (60 percent of total calories from fat) and relatively high in sugar (17.6 percent of total calories), at the end of the study, the mice whose dietary fat came mostly from soybean oil weighed the most, while the mice who were fed mostly fish oil weighed the least. In order from highest to lowest body weight, the oils that made up most of the diet were: soybean, palm, lard, canola, safflower, perilla, and fish oil.[22] Yes, you read that correctly: soybean oil—one of the omega-6 "vegetable oils" we've been encouraged to eat, made mice *fatter than lard did*! Perilla and fish oil, which are high in omega-3s, made mice the leanest.

But it gets even worse. Among the different fats tested, the ones highest in omega-6 linoleic acid were positively associated with higher blood-glucose levels—meaning the more linoleic acid the mice ate, the higher their blood sugar. After being given a large dose of sugar, the mice that were fed safflower oil (made up of a whopping 78 percent linoleic acid) had the highest glucose area under the curve, while the mice that were fed fish oil had the lowest. This suggests that compared to a diet high in omega-6 fats, a diet high in long-chain omega-3s (EPA and DHA) may help to mitigate weight gain and blood-sugar elevations caused by a diet high in sugar.

These noteworthy findings have been replicated in other studies. For example, rats fed fish oil had less total body fat, less intra-abdominal (visceral) fat, and less insulin resistance than those fed corn oil or lard.[23] Mouse studies show that long-chain omega-3 fats increase fat burning inside fat cells, and inhibit fat-cell growth and proliferation.[24,25,26,27] In other words, while omega-6-heavy oils contribute to obesity and higher blood sugar, long-chain omega-3s are *anti*-obesogenic.

FAMILY TREE OF FAT

In case you thought this was all about *you*, let's take a minute to talk about your children and grandchildren. The number of fat cells an individual has is determined during childhood and adolescence.[28] Large numbers of animal studies clearly show that omega-6 fats increase the formation of fully developed fat cells from preadipocytes (fat cell precursors), leading to increased fat accumulation, whereas omega-3 fats have the opposite effect.[29,30,31] Pregnant and breastfeeding mice fed omega-3 ALA even in the presence of omega-6 had offspring with lower total body weight, lower body fat, and smaller individual fat cells compared to offspring from mice fed a high-omega-6 diet without ALA.[32]

Okay, that's good to know . . . for mice. What about in humans? In humans, mothers with high blood levels of omega-6 had children with increased body fat at four and six years of age, whereas higher maternal omega-3 levels were correlated with greater lean mass.[33] So mothers with high omega-6 levels compared to omega-3 during pregnancy will simply have fatter children than women with lower omega-6-to-3 ratios.

In the previous chapter, we detailed how a pregnant woman's omega-6 and omega-3 intake can influence her child's health—especially mental health—into adolescence and even later in life. It seems the same is true for setting children up for an easier time maintaining a healthy weight or for putting them on the path to fight their own bodies' tendency to hoard fat. A study called Project Viva showed that a higher omega-6-to-3 ratio in the maternal diet and in cord blood correlates with increased child obesity.[34] When moms have more omega-3 fats in their bodies, and these fats are passed along to their babies, the babies are less likely to be overweight during childhood. If you're pregnant, or thinking about becoming pregnant, please be sure to determine your omega-3 status to give your child the best start he or she can get toward lifelong metabolic heath.

It's often said that obesity is genetic or that it runs in families. The things that really run in families are dietary and lifestyle habits, so it's true that there's a familial aspect to it, but there doesn't appear to be an obesity gene. However, **the stage is set in the womb, driven by the good fats and bad fats in Mom's diet, so that regardless of what kind of diet you follow now, your**

literal formative months may have made it harder or easier to maintain a healthy weight as an adult.

Remember, though, you don't need to worry so much about consuming excessive omega-6 from whole, unprocessed foods, such as nuts and seeds, where these fragile fatty acids are protected by antioxidants and other phytonutrients that keep them from being damaged by rancidity and oxidation. The omega-6s you want to avoid are the ones in liquid oils and the processed foods that contain these oils: soybean, corn, safflower, cottonseed, and sunflower.

Read the labels at the supermarket, and you'll find these oils in just about everything, but some of the worst offenders are salad dressings, mayonnaise, margarine, and imitation butters made from plant oils, frosting, crackers, cookies, cakes (almost all baked goods, in fact), peanut butter, microwave meals, and more.

MARINE OMEGA-3S AND FAT LOSS

If you've ever struggled to lose weight, or know someone who has, then you know it's not as easy as the experts make it sound. Plenty of people dutifully follow the often-parroted advice to "eat less and move more," to no avail. They mercilessly remove every visible molecule of fat from their food and spend precious hours whittling away time on a treadmill or elliptical machine only to see little to no change in their weight or shape. "Frustrating" is an understatement.

People who face an uphill battle to lose weight can use every bit of help they can get. **Considering the role of omega-3 fats in improving insulin sensitivity and reducing inflammation, it shouldn't come as much of a surprise that these wondrous molecules can be an ace in the hole for fat loss.** Many animal studies have found greater lean-mass gains (muscle, bone, connective tissue), lower fat-mass and intra-abdominal fat gains, increased insulin sensitivity, and increased metabolic rate with diets higher in fish oil compared to other types of fats (such as vegetable oils, olive oil, lard, and beef tallow).[35,36,37] These results occurred despite each of the fats providing the same number of calories—meaning, when it comes to weight loss, the *type* of fat you eat is just as important, or maybe even *more* important—than the total amount. Even when added as *extra* calories in addition to a diet already high in saturated fat and omega-6 fats, omega-3 fish oils help to reduce the growth of fat cells and the deposition of dangerous visceral fat.[38]

In a study that followed obese women eating a very low calorie diet, subjects who took fish-oil supplements experienced greater weight loss and larger reductions in body mass index and hip circumference compared to subjects who followed the same diet but did not take fish oil.[39] **Omega-3s seem to *boost your body's overall efficiency at fat burning*. It's not just the overall metabolism that runs better; it's the burning of *fats*, specifically.**

Remember, if you want to lose body fat, then that's what you've got to burn—*fat*. It does no good to burn more carbohydrates. The study authors concluded, "The results suggest that EPA and DHA enhance weight loss in obese females treated by very low-calorie diet. DHA, more than EPA, seems to be the active component."[40] The part of this that matters in the real world: adding EPA and DHA to low-calorie diets may help people lose more fat than dieting alone, and of the specific compounds that are responsible for this effect, DHA is the most powerful.

What about if you're already healthy? Can omega-3 fats still be of benefit for helping to maintain a healthy body weight? *Even with no change to your diet or exercise habits*, consuming more marine omega-3s can *still* have a beneficial effect on your body composition. And whereas the omega-3s offer benefits, omega-6s actually have *adverse* effects.

When it comes to improving your health, losing "weight" is not as important as losing *fat*. So it's better to measure body-fat percentage than it is to measure scale weight. Marine oils win here, too! Again, the absolute changes were small, but in one study, subjects who took fish oil lost body fat, while subjects taking safflower oil *gained* it. Resting metabolic rate (the amount of energy, or calories, your body burns even while you're lying around doing nothing) was increased in the fish-oil group but decreased in the safflower-oil group. Fish oil added to weight-loss diets has been found to cause greater reductions in weight and waist circumference than the same diet without fish oil.[41]

EPA and DHA increase fat burning and decrease fat building—a win-win for anyone trying to get rid of stubborn body fat.[42] In order to reduce body fat—whether it's on your hips and thighs, or in and around your internal organs, give yourself a fat fix: less omega-6, more omega-3.

DHA: Your "Pacemaker" of Metabolism

One of the keys to maintaining a healthy weight is having a high metabolic rate. After all, most exercise doesn't come close to the energy your body expends just to keep you alive. If you could find a way to adjust this internal "thermostat," then you'd burn more calories around the clock, even when you're *not* exercising. It's not easy to accomplish this, but one way that might be effective is raising the body's concentration of DHA.

Long-chain omega-3 fats, particularly DHA, are the main determinants of basal metabolic rate (the temperature your body's thermostat is set to).[43] Several years ago, biologists proposed the idea that cell membranes act like pacemakers for metabolic rate. They observed that warm-blooded mammals and birds have much higher basal metabolic rates than those of similar sized cold-blooded reptiles, amphibians, and fish. They discovered that this is due to a greater amount of polyunsaturated fats in cell membranes: small mammals have greater cell-membrane polyunsaturated fat content compared to the cold-blooded animals.

They also discovered that the degree of unsaturation of fats in mammalian cell membranes relates to body-mass index (i.e., compared to small mammals, larger mammals have less omega-3 in their cell membranes). DHA, in particular, acts like a cellular energizer: the highest concentrations of DHA are found in cell membranes of organs and tissues involved in very fast-paced or nonstop activity, such as in hummingbird wings, and in the hearts, brains, and sperm cells (which have to swim far and fast for survival) of numerous animals.[44]

With this in mind, increasing the unsaturated fat content of your cell membranes—especially with omega-3s—increases the metabolic activity of proteins bound to those membranes, which contribute to at least 50 percent of the overall basal metabolic rate. Perhaps this explains why studies show omega-3 supplements increase basal metabolic rate. Imagine that: increasing the amount of energy your body uses *even while you're relaxing*, just by getting a healthy amount of omega-3s in your diet. We weren't kidding when we said how important cell membranes are!

These membrane-bound proteins are affected by the degree of unsaturation of the fats in the cell membrane. They are less active when cell membranes contain higher amounts of saturated and monounsaturated fats, as well as cholesterol. All these elements are required for healthy cell-membrane function; it's only when they're in the wrong proportions that things go awry and cellular function—including the burning of fat—is compromised. If you have a dog or cat, maybe you go out of your way to feed him high-quality food to make sure he stays healthy. Do the same for your cell membranes: feed them plenty of good omega-3s. With the increased metabolic rate this might cause, your waistline will thank you.

Marine Omega-3s and Muscle Gains: More Muscle, More Fat Burning

Another prime way to increase your basal metabolic rate is to increase the amount of muscle mass you carry. Muscle tissue is "metabolically expensive." It requires energy just to *exist*, let alone to perform exercise, when it requires even more energy. And when you read "requires energy," think *burns fat*. Is there a role for omega-3 fats in helping to increase muscle mass? Yes! When cell membranes contain greater amounts of long-chain omega-3s, your body's resting metabolic rate increases, as does protein synthesis—and if you want to build muscle, you've got to synthesize proteins.[45]

There are a wide variety of proteins embedded within your cell membranes to help transport nutrients (including sodium, calcium, glucose, and amino acids, just to name a few) into and out of the cell. Having more omega-3s in your cell membranes makes these processes work better and faster,[46] because having the right amount of omega-3s in your cell membranes gives the membranes the proper shape. And if your cell membranes *don't* have the proper shape, then these embedded proteins might not have the right shape or orientation, either. And when a protein has the wrong shape or orientation, it doesn't work the way it was designed to.

AGING: MAINTAINING MUSCLE MASS

The natural loss of muscle mass that occurs during the normal aging process—called *sarcopenia*—is a significant health problem. It reduces strength and mobility, increases the risk of falls, reduces overall quality of life, and may even lead to premature death.[47] In middle-aged individuals, muscle mass declines by a rate of approximately 0.5 to 1 percent per year, with a corresponding loss of muscle *function* of 2 to 3 percent per year.[48] This might not sound like much, but think about it: when you're 60 years old, you could be *30 percent weaker* than you were when you were 50. That could have major implications for your ability to live independently. Forget doing a bench press or lifting heavy weights: would you still be able to carry heavy grocery bags or walk up a few flights of stairs? Unless you're a professional bodybuilder, building and maintaining muscle tissue has nothing to do with vanity and everything to do with maintaining your long-term health and mobility.

Sarcopenia is primarily attributed to something called "anabolic resistance." Anabolism is the technical word for "building things up." (Think of testosterone—it's an *anabolic* hormone, because it contributes to the building up of muscle mass.) Anabolic *resistance* is when the body has a lower response to factors that would normally cause anabolism, such as insulin and amino acids, as well as testosterone. As you age, your body doesn't respond as strongly to these factors as it did when you were younger. This has a lot to do with hormonal changes during aging, but fats also have an effect. Omega-3 supplementation has been shown to increase the anabolic response to amino acids and insulin, which might help stave off this frailty as you age.

Animals given omega-3 supplementation have an increase in whole-body protein synthesis and activation of anabolic-signaling proteins in muscle when administered insulin and amino acids.[49] The phrase "whole-body protein synthesis" is key. You probably first think of muscles when you hear the word "protein," and it's true that muscles are made from protein, but so are bones, hair, skin, nails, joints, tendons, and ligaments—and that's just the short list!

The antibodies and white blood cells the immune system uses to fight off infections are also made from proteins, and maybe this is why elderly people, with their reduced protein synthesis, are at greater risk for colds, flu, and other infectious illnesses. Omega-3s have a long history of preventing loss of muscle mass and increasing muscle growth and strength in a wide variety of clinical settings, testing cancer, burns, rheumatoid arthritis, and more.[50,51,52,53,54]

Omega-3 fats also help to preserve muscle tissue on two fronts: they increase the building of muscle while also reducing muscle breakdown.[55] Unlike omega-6 fats, which induce inflammation and signal the body to store fat—including dangerous fat stored in the liver—omega-3s *reduce* fat accumulation in the liver, as well as in muscles.[56,57,58] Preventing fat accumulation in muscles might be one of the ways omega-3s reduce the loss of muscle strength with aging.

Other mechanisms include an increase in mitochondrial biogenesis, content, and function.[59] Recall from Chapter 6 that mitochondria are the energy generators of ATP inside your cells.

They are the actual sites where molecules from the foods you eat are converted into energy. And because your muscles need energy to give them strength and power, they're loaded with mitochondria. A single muscle cell can contain thousands. You might say that when it comes to aging, you're only as old as your mitochondria.

Clearly, then, in order to age gracefully and with your mental capacity fully intact, you want to support healthy mitochondrial function. Adequate omega-3s do just that. Omega-3s stimulate mitochondrial biogenesis (the making of new mitochondria) and support healthy mitochondrial function. One study found that supplementation with 2 grams of fish oil per day enhanced the effects of strength training in elderly women within just three months by improving muscle strength and functional capacity.[60] The authors suggested that omega-3s may lead to faster muscle contraction via improved cell-membrane function and faster nerve-impulse transmission, the latter powered in part by mito-chondria. It's never too late to build muscle, and no one is too old or too "senior" a citizen to start a strength training program. Find a qualified trainer to work with, start lifting weights . . . **and take your fish or krill oil.**

Marine Omega-3s May Improve Your Energy, Reduce Fatigue, and Increase Your Exercise Capacity

The benefits of omega-3s don't stop at preserving muscle mass and supporting the growth of new muscle tissue. Omega-3s also improve what happens when you *use* those muscles. EPA and DHA have been found to improve oxygen efficiency in humans during exercise. In one study looking at 16 well-trained cyclists, com-pared to olive oil, a daily dose of 3.2 grams of omega-3 for eight weeks resulted in lowered heart rate and reduced whole-body oxy-gen consumption during exercise.[61] The less oxygen consumed during exercise, the more efficient an athlete's body is, so this is a good thing.

Same thing with heart rate: in healthy people, the lower the heart rate during a period of exertion, the stronger the heart muscle is—so it can pump blood more powerfully with each contraction, and therefore requires fewer contractions to get the job done. Keep in mind, though, that this applies to *healthy* people. Older people, or those with compromised cardiovascular function, may have lower heart rates because their heart muscle is weakened. The authors concluded, "This study indicates that fish oil may act within the healthy heart and skeletal muscle to reduce both whole-body and myocardial oxygen demand during exercise, without a decrement in performance."

Those last few words are key: *no decrement in performance* means they were able to generate the same amount of power and speed while consuming less oxygen and with a lower heart rate. In other words, their bodies had become more efficient. Think of it like taking a car with a run-of-the-mill engine and swapping out that engine for a turbocharged Porsche V8. The regular engine gets the job done, but the improved one gets better mileage, runs more smoothly, and makes for a superior driving experience.

Not only were these athletes' bodies more efficient with the marine-oil supplementation, but their own ratings of *perceived* exertion regarding their whole bodies, and chests specifically, were significantly improved. What this means is that while they were exercising, they felt like they were exerting themselves less even though they were doing the same amount of work. A lower perceived rate of exertion can help trained athletes and beginners alike work longer and harder before feeling fatigued, which could potentially lead to better results, such as improved speed, strength, or endurance.

Table 7.1 is a summary of the beneficial effects that long-chain marine omega-3s can have for athletic performance.

Table 7.1: Benefits of Long-Chain Marine Omega-3s for Weight Loss and Muscle Gains

Decreased:	Increased:
• Fat synthesis and fat mass • Hunger (reduced caloric intake and improved satiety after meals) • Muscle loss • Exercise-induced fatigue • Inflamed fat tissue • Cortisol levels (less stress-induced weight gain) • Ectopic fat accumulation (accumulation of intramuscular fat and visceral fat, especially in your liver)	• Fat burning (at rest, during exercise, and after a sugar load) • Lean mass • Muscle growth and strength • Metabolic rate at rest and during exercise • Exercise capacity and performance • Mitochondrial biogenesis and function

Most adults should consume at least 2 grams of combined EPA and DHA per day in order to provide enough omega-3s for healthy cell membranes, to support increased fat burning, and to prevent loss of muscle mass. For maximal effects on gaining muscle mass and strength, older adults may need higher amounts—around 3 to 4 grams per day.

Summary

- Subcutaneous fat (the fat just beneath our skin, the stuff we all like to avoid) is far less dangerous than visceral fat, the fat that can collect around your organs.

- This kind of stored fat frequently becomes inflamed so that it sends incorrect signals to your body (e.g., causing blood vessels to constrict) or fails to send correct signals (e.g., to trigger resolvins and protectins to combat the inflammation).

- Industrial seed oils (omega-6s) tend to cause inflammation, while GLA, oleic acid, and omega-3 fats decrease it.

- Our bodies' ability to process these fats is determined in utero; if we are given high levels of industrial seed oils without high levels of DHA to combat them, we will have trouble maintaining healthy body weight as we grow and age.

- Omega-3s, particularly DHA, tell your body to burn more fat.

- Sarcopenia, the process of muscular degeneration with age, can be offset with sufficient omega-3 intake, as these help to preserve muscle tissue on two fronts: they increase the building of muscle while also reducing muscle breakdown. They also help maintain mitochondrial function.

CHAPTER 8

FISH OIL AND BEYOND: GUIDE TO LESSER-KNOWN OILS AND SUPPLEMENTS

We've been emphasizing throughout this book that decreasing your omega-6 intake and increasing your intake of omega-3 fats—especially EPA and DHA—are simple and highly effective steps you can take to improve multiple aspects of your health. But there are other important fats we haven't yet discussed, as there's definitely more to good fats than just fish oil. Whether you're already healthy and looking to stay that way, or you're dealing with a specific condition that might respond to a change in the fats you consume, getting the right mix of fats can tip things in your favor. Some health conditions may respond to specific kinds of fats not typically found in the foods you consume most of the time, so we'll show you what these fats are, and how to take them.

Converting Crucial Fats from Omega-3 and Omega-6

In order for the "parent" omega-3 and omega-6 fats to convert into longer-chain fats, they require helper molecules called enzymes. As you can see from Figure 8.1, delta-6 desaturase (D6D) is the enzyme required to set these conversions in motion; it's the first domino to get knocked over, and it makes all the ones after it fall down too.

Insulin stimulates D6D—that is, it signals your body to make and use this enzyme—thus, higher levels of insulin reduce levels of LA, because LA starts moving through the conversion process. On the other hand, *low* levels of insulin can *reduce* the activity of D6D, leaving LA to accumulate, because without the help of this enzyme, LA cannot start making its way down the conversion pathway. Without sufficient D6D activity, your body can't convert the parent omega-6 and omega-3s into the other types of fatty acids that come from them, such as gamma-linolenic acid (GLA), dihomo-gamma linolenic acid (DGLA), and arachidonic acid (formed from LA), or EPA and DHA (formed from ALA).[1]

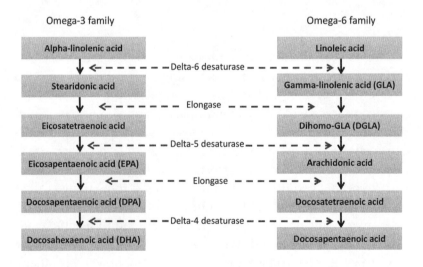

Figure 8.1: The Elongation of Omega-3 and Omega-6 Fats[2]

As parent omega-6 and omega-3 fats move through their conversion process, they require different enzymes—different dominoes. Delta-5-desaturase (D5D) is the next domino. The Dutch Cohort study on Diabetes and Atherosclerosis Maastricht (CoDAM) found a lower D5D activity in those with type 2 diabetes compared to nondiabetics.[3] Other studies have found that not only do high insulin levels correlate with lower D5D activity, but they also correlate with higher activity of D6D.[4,5,6] So chronically elevated insulin levels *increase* the activity of the first enzyme in this pathway, while *decreasing* activity of one that comes later.[7] This creates a kind of logjam in the system.

In looking specifically at the omega-3 side of this pathway, increased activity of D6D reduces levels of ALA, since ALA starts moving through the process, but with *decreased* activity of D5D, the crucial fats that come later on—EPA and DHA—don't get produced. For this reason, individuals with insulin resistance are particularly susceptible to deficiencies in EPA and DHA. Even if you're not diabetic, you should note that insulin resistance is widely underdiagnosed; pathologist Joseph Kraft, M.D., designed a sensitive insulin-resistance test that suggests around 75 percent of the adult population are insulin resistant.

How do you fix this? The answer depends on which situation applies: too much insulin, or too little. Type 1 diabetics have impaired activity of both D6D and D5D, which is restored to normal levels by insulin therapy.[8] But type 2 diabetics and the 75 percent of the population with insulin resistance would likely benefit from EPA and DHA. Table 8.1 is a summary of the effects of insulin resistance on omega-6 and omega-3 metabolism.

Table 8.1: The Effects of Hyperinsulinemia/Insulin Resistance on Omega-6 and Omega-3 Metabolism

Omega-3	Omega-6
Insulin stimulates D6D leading to • Low ALA • High stearidonic and eicosatetraenoic acid	Insulin stimulates D6D leading to • Low LA • High GLA • High DGLA
Insulin resistance inhibits D5D leading to • Low EPA • Low DHA	Insulin resistance inhibits D5D leading to • Low AA

Insulin isn't the only hormone that affects the activity of these fat-converting enzymes. Glucagon, adrenaline, cortisol, and aldosterone are just a handful of the other hormones that influence these biochemical processes.[9] Diets very low in sodium (salt) increase adrenaline and aldosterone, and these hormones *reduce* activity of D6D and D5D. For this reason, low-salt diets increase the need for EPA and DHA due to the reduced desaturase enzyme activities. Another extremely common hormonal issue these days, one that interferes with conversion of the parent omega-6 and omega-3 fats into their derivatives, is hypothyroidism. Thyroid hormone is required for proper activity of D6D and D5D, so individuals with suboptimal thyroid hormone levels may benefit from consuming more EPA and DHA or taking good-quality supplements.[10]

And remember, LA and ALA *compete* for the conversion enzymes, and the more omega-6 LA in your diet, the more it will crowd out omega-3 ALA for use of those enzymes. To give you some numbers here, increasing LA intake from 15 to 30 grams per day decreases the conversion of ALA into EPA and DHA by a whopping 40 percent.[11] To translate that to something meaningful at the dinner table, a single generous serving of salad dressing could account for 15 grams of linoleic acid all by itself! High insulin levels, low thyroid hormone levels, and consumption of omega-6 and trans fats: it's no wonder so many millions of people suffer the effects of omega-3 deficiencies.

MEDIUM-CHAIN TRIGLYCERIDES

Medium-chain triglycerides (MCTs) are saturated fats that are 6 to 12 carbons in length,[12] based on the number of carbon atoms in the molecule. For example, butyric acid (found in butter) has just 4 carbon atoms and is considered a *short*-chain fatty acid, and oleic acid (found in olive oil and lard) has 18 carbon atoms and is considered a *long*-chain fatty acid. The foods you are probably most familiar with that are sources of MCTs are coconut oil, Roquefort cheese, and palm-kernel oil (which is used mostly in chocolates, candies, and other confections).

MCTs are considered ideal for weight loss compared to longer-chain fats because they're not metabolized the same way as other fats. Other fats pass from the small intestine into the lymphatic system and then into the bloodstream, where they can be delivered to cells to be used as fuel right away, or stored in fat cells for use at another time. Contrast this with MCTs, which pass from your small intestine directly to your liver, which either uses them for fuel or converts them into ketones, which are another kind of fuel other cells can use. Because of this difference, it's less likely that fats containing MCTs will be stored as body fat compared to other fats.

Additionally, the rapid conversion of MCTs into fuel leads to enhanced satiety and decreased food intake, which may be why MCTs have been shown to be less obesity-inducing compared to long-chain saturated fats.[13] A meta-analysis of thirteen randomized controlled trials found that compared to long-chain fats, MCTs decrease body weight, waist circumference, hip circumference, total body fat, and, perhaps most important, visceral fat.[14]

So if any fat can be said to be good for *losing* fat, it's MCTs. This is why coconut oil has become so popular recently. You can also find pure MCT oils as a supplement in health-food stores; some people enjoy adding a spoonful or two of coconut oil or MCT oil to their morning coffee or tea for a quick energy boost on top of the caffeine.

Obese people often have impaired fat burning of long-chain saturated fats. That is, they don't "burn" long-chain saturated fats and get energy from them as effectively as leaner people do. The same doesn't hold true for MCTs, though.[15] Consuming MCTs, at least compared to long-chain saturated fats, results in greater energy use at the cellular level after meals, and greater energy use means "burning more calories" *even if you're not exercising.* This doesn't mean you can be a couch potato and expect to look like dynamite by simply eating more MCTs, but it might mean that when you're already following a healthy diet and getting a good amount of physical activity, MCTs can be an extra tool in the toolbox—a little ace up your sleeve for boosting your fat burning even more.

Coconut Oil

Pure MCT oil isn't suitable for cooking, as it contains mostly caprylic and capric acids, both of which have low smoke points. Coconut oil, on the other hand, is great for cooking, because about 50 percent of its fat content is an MCT called lauric acid, which has a high smoke point, suitable for frying and sautéing.

Aside from a higher smoke point, another thing coconut oil and other high-lauric-acid oils have going for them as cooking oils is that they're low in fragile, unstable unsaturated fats and are therefore less likely to oxidize and turn rancid—and therefore harmful—when heated. So, if you're following a weight-loss plan but still want to enjoy the flavor and satiety dietary fat offers, coconut oil is a good option for cooking compared to the saturated fats in butter or lard, and definitely compared to the fats in soybean and corn oils. Compared to soybean oil, coconut oil has been shown to promote abdominal fat loss in humans.[16] In a small study of 20 obese but otherwise healthy individuals, virgin coconut oil caused a 1-inch reduction in waist circumference in just one week.[17] It appears that coconut oil shares some of the anti-obesogenic properties of the traditional MCTs.

Fat Oxidation Rates

Consuming fats with higher oxidation rates may lead to less weight gain, due to reduced fat storage and enhanced fat burning for energy. Lauric acid is one of the most highly oxidized fats in humans, which may explain why coconut oil seems to be such a good fat for weight loss.[18,19] Unsaturated fats and long-chain saturated fats have lower oxidation rates, though long-chain unsaturated fats are easier to metabolize and thus oxidized at a higher rate compared to long-chain saturated fats.[20] Within the category of saturated fats, the oxidation rate decreases with *increased* chain length—that is, the longer the carbon chain of a saturated fat, the *lower* the oxidation rate. In terms of oxidation rate: caprylic acid (8 carbons) > lauric acid (12 carbons) > myristic acid (14 carbons) > palmitic acid (16 carbons) > stearic acid (18 carbons). Thus, owing to their higher oxidation rates, medium-chain saturated fats may be better for weight loss than longer-chain fats.[21,22] One animal study showed that animals given MCTs (with their high oxidation rates) via parenteral nutrition (intravenous feeding) had increased daily energy expenditure and just one-third the weight gain of animals given long-chain fats.[23]

What does this mean to you in the real world when it comes time to eat? Well, if you're looking to lose body fat while still maintaining your health, you might want to cut the fat off your steak and use a little coconut oil instead. Keep in mind, of course, that fat loss depends on many factors besides the oxidation rate of a fat. Choosing to get more of your dietary fat from MCTs rather than from beef or pork fat is just a little "hack" to stack the deck in your favor.

If your goal is to lose fat, here are the good, better, and best choices for which fats to eat, and also the ones you should avoid as much as possible. For better fat-loss results, try to incorporate foods in the better and best columns:

Avoid	Good	Better	Best
Trans fats	LA from whole foods (e.g., nuts and seeds)	Omega-3s Marine sources (EPA and DHA from seafood) Plant sources (ALA from nuts, seeds, and grass-fed meat and eggs)	Medium-chain triglycerides
Industrial seed oils (soybean, corn, cottonseed, safflower oils)	Palm oil	Oleic acid (olive oil, macadamia nuts, avocado)	Coconut oil

Note that this applies mainly to individuals who consume a moderate-to-high amount of carbohydrates. Individuals following low-carbohydrate diets may have different results.

Some of the MCT-oil products you see in stores are purified oils that contain only fats with 8 carbons, but less expensive versions that don't convert to ketones as easily are mixtures of C8 and C10 fats. Some manufacturers now produce MCT oils that contain up to 30 percent lauric acid (a fat with 12 carbons, found predominantly in coconut oil) because this raises the smoke point, making it better suited for cooking than regular MCT oil. MCT oils formulated to contain lauric acid tend to have fewer of the unpleasant side-effects some people experience from consuming large amounts of regular MCT oil, such as upset stomach or loose stools.[24]

Other uses for MCT oil include adding some to your coffee or tea for a ketone boost or using it in homemade salad dressing. Just don't make it all out of MCT oil; use mostly extra-virgin olive oil or avocado oil and replace a little of that with MCT oil. There's no need to supplement with MCT oil or coconut oil, but you can use coconut oil and high-lauric-acid MCT oils for cooking and baking, or use coconut oil as a skin moisturizer.

What Does It All Mean?

Cutting back on refined carbohydrates is a great strategy for weight loss, but for people who can't imagine life without bread, the *type* of fat they eat will help them offset a little carb indulgence. And paying attention to the kinds of fat you eat is particularly important for those with type 2 diabetes or insulin resistance. For these individuals, consuming foods with more omega-3s (seafood and flax), MCTs (coconut oil) and monounsaturated fats (avocados, nuts, olive oil) may facilitate greater fat loss and improvement in insulin sensitivity compared to foods that contain trans fats, industrial seed oils, and full-fat dairy (butter, cheese, cream, milk).

Monounsaturated fats, MCTs, and omega-3s (especially EPA and DHA) are a dietary "dream team" when it comes to losing body fat, preserving muscle mass, and building even more lean muscle. These fats send your body messages to let go of excess fat, hold on to precious muscle, and keep your metabolism humming along, whether you're in the middle of a workout or just relaxing.

On the other hand, vegetable oils high in omega-6 set in motion the perfect storm for gaining body fat and *hanging onto that fat*, no matter how hard you work to get rid of it. So instead of reaching for a burger from a corn-fed cow, favor meat from grass-fed and pastured animals, and make wild-caught seafood a bigger part of your diet. The critically important omega-3s are fats you can definitely feel good about eating.

Supplements: Pushing through the Overwhelm

We believe that whole foods are always the best sources of nutrients, and in Chapter 9, we'll walk you through the good food fats to choose and the bad food fats to avoid. But we also understand that it's not easy to consume as much healthy toxin-free seafood as you might need to get a "therapeutic dose" of DHA and EPA—enough to make a significant impact on a specific condition, and your budget might not allow for a diet consisting exclusively of grass-fed meats, wild game, and other foods richer in DHA and EPA. Plus, if you've been following a conventional Western diet for most of your life, you might have to first dig yourself out of the omega-6 hole, so to speak—to consume extra omega-3s in order to establish a better balance of fats in your body before decreasing your dose down to an everyday maintenance level.

With these issues in mind, it might be nearly impossible for you to get enough omega-3s solely through whole foods. This is where supplementation comes in. We understand that sorting through the overload of capsules, bottles, powders, and pills at the store can be so overwhelming that no one could blame you for giving up and walking out empty-handed. And while we've written extensively about the detrimental changes in the modern food supply that have wreaked havoc on your health, there are some aspects of modern food technology that can serve your best interests. Marine oils (fish, krill, and algal oil) and other fatty-acid supplements are among them.

Fish Oil

Since fish oil is the most economical supplemental source of DHA and EPA, let's start there. It is important to be wary of mass-marketed fish oils that come with an extremely low price tag. Improperly manufactured and stored fish oils will likely cause you more harm than good. Remember, these fats are highly unsaturated, so they're easily oxidized, and some less-than-reputable brands might not even contain the full amounts of EPA and DHA claimed on their labels.[25] Since heat and light are two of the factors that damage these fragile oils, it's a good idea to store fish oil in the refrigerator and it might be even better to store it in the freezer. (Pure fish oil won't freeze.) We recommend taking omega-3s with your largest meal of the day in order to reduce the mild gastrointestinal discomfort that might result, as well as the "fishy burps" some people experience.

As for dosing, the U.S. FDA considers 3 grams of combined EPA and DHA per day to be safe. When eating fish, you should be selective about where your fish oil comes from because not all fish are created equal. Certain fish may have levels of mercury and other contaminants high enough to outweigh the benefits you might get from taking fish oil derived from them. Salmon are lower in these contaminants than other fish, but fish oil supplements derived from smaller fish and other aquatic life lower down on the marine food chain (such as sardines, anchovies, or krill) are even safer.[26]

But as far as supplements go, the good news is that regardless of what type of fish oil you take, the production of this kind of oil requires extensive processing and purification, including distillation at a relatively high temperature. This refinement removes heavy metals and also reduces a number of persistent organic pollutants.[27] As a result, concern about heavy metals and other pollutants in fish and other seafood is a more important issue when purchasing these foods to eat rather than the purified oils. On the other hand, this purification process must be handled carefully so as not to damage these highly fragile oils, so make sure you are using a reputable source, which may not necessarily be the cheapest.

Fish Oil: Does Formulation Matter?

In their natural state, EPA and DHA are bound in triglycerides, for just as we store our fat with triglycerides, so too do fish. Prescription fish oils, on the other hand, typically contain EPA and DHA bound in another kind of molecule called an ethyl ester. Some manufacturers produce fish oils that have been restored to the triglyceride form, referred to as re-esterified TAG, or rTAG. Although both forms are effective for increasing the omega-3 index (the amount of omega-3s in red blood cells), the rTAG form gets the job done a bit better, so look for fish oils produced by manufacturers who take this extra step.[28,29,30]

A Word of Caution on Heavily Refined Omega-3 Oils

As you learned in Chapters 2 and 3, the industrial refinement of food may have unintended consequences. In the case of trans fat, it was a health catastrophe on a global scale, with the true extent of damage not known until nearly a century later. When you source your marine fats naturally (i.e., by eating fish rather than supplements) your EPA and DHA come with many other complex fatty acids and nutrients, which have additional benefits, including some we may not yet fully understand. Heavy refinement of omega-3 oils may alter or destroy these naturally occurring compounds in ways we cannot anticipate, but we don't want to make the same overindustrializing mistake twice. **We recommend choosing supplements that have undergone only minimal and careful processing.**

Guidelines for supplementing with fish oil:

1. Store in the refrigerator or freezer

2. Keep away from light

3. Take with a meal

4. Avoid consuming with iron-rich foods, as iron may oxidize omega-3 PUFAs in the acidic environment of the stomach

5. The optimal dose of combined EPA and DHA for most people is 3 to 4 grams per day

Krill Oil

Krill, tiny crustaceans that resemble shrimp, are found in oceans around the globe. The most abundant species of krill, *Euphasia superba*, are found only in the cold Southern Ocean that surrounds the continent Antarctica. Known as Antarctic Krill, this unique species feeds on microalgae in swarms so large that they can be seen from outer space.[31] Krill are located at the near-bottom of the food chain, which in combination with living in a very clean environment, means they are virtually free from many of the harmful contaminants found in larger marine species.

Compared to other forms of omega-3 supplements, krill oil has the highest absorption rate of the omega-3s EPA and DHA into tissue.[32] The EPA and DHA in krill oil are largely bound to phospholipids, an important component of cell membranes. These phospholipids are digested by your body differently—and better—than the fish oils found in ethyl ester or triglyceride form; recent research has shown that the delivery of fatty acids like DHA and arachidonic acid into the brain and tissue is directly dependent on the fatty acids being in phospholipid form.[33,34,35]

Besides containing an efficient form of both EPA and DHA, krill contains many other beneficial nutrients, including astaxanthin. Astaxanthin is a powerful antioxidant that is responsible for the pink color found in krill, salmon, and even flamingos. It's commonly referred to as the "king of antioxidants," and for good reason: studies have suggested that astaxanthin is 6,000 times more potent an antioxidant than Vitamin C, 550 times more potent than Vitamin E, and 40 times more potent than beta-carotene.[36]

In addition to astaxanthin, krill oil also contains a large dose of choline at 55 to 75 mg of choline per gram of krill oil. Choline is an essential nutrient for a diverse array of critical bodily functions. Like EPA and DHA, the choline in krill is bound to phospholipids, making them phosphatidylcholine—a highly absorbable form of this valuable and difficult-to-obtain nutrient. Research suggests that phosphatidylcholine can support liver health and prevent the progression of nonalcoholic fatty liver disease (NAFLD).[37] In addition, for the brain to effectively absorb omega-3 fatty acids, it must pass through a specific transport molecule known as Mfsd2A.[38,39,40] This process requires that fatty acids are bound to lysophosphatidylcholine.

(You can get your phosphatidylcholine as supplemental lecithin, derived from either soy or sunflower, but note that in lecithin, the fats are omega-6, rather than long-chain EPA or DHA, so you would be without those additional benefits).

The phospholipids in krill are fragile structures, so to maintain the integrity of the precious omega-3 oil, it must be gently extracted using natural ethanol, water, and a low-heat process. Because of this gentle and natural extraction process, as well as the absence of many of the harmful contaminants found in the ocean, **krill oil is closer to a clean, whole food than any other processed fish oil.**

Concerns about Krill Sustainability

How sustainable is the krill-fishing industry in their frigid Arctic home? Since krill are a primary food source for whales, many have expressed concerns that harvesting krill is killing the whales. The marine ecosystem is very delicate, so this is a legitimate concern that responsible krill-oil manufacturers have gone to great lengths to respect. In 1982, as part of the Antarctica Treaty System, the Convention on the Conservation of Antarctic Marine Living Resources (CCAMLR) was established, largely due to concerns about krill fisheries in the region.

The CCAMLR regulates krill fisheries, helping to prevent any adverse impacts on the fragile Antarctic ecosystem. Some krill-oil fisheries have even taken their sustainability efforts further, certifying themselves under the prestigious Marine Stewardship Council (MSC), an organization dedicated to the preservation of Earth's oceans. The MSC website states, "The best available science from CCAMLR suggests that krill fishing is at such a low level that penguins and marine mammals, which also consume krill in large quantities, are not negatively impacted by fishing activity."[41]

When it comes to health benefits, krill oil has more advantages over other omega-3 oils. For example, krill oil beats fish oil for maximum efficacy in terms of improving blood lipids and reducing inflammation and oxidative stress. According to one study, EPA and DHA from krill oil could achieve similar benefits to fish oil at about 60 percent of the dose,[42] meaning that you could take a lower dose but have the same effects, since your body assimilates and incorporates krill oil more efficiently than fish oil.

With specific regard to reaching your brain, the bioavailability of omega-3s from krill may be twice as high as that of traditional fish oil,[43] though fish oil may lead to higher general levels of DHA compared to krill oil, which may be beneficial in certain situations, such as for people looking to lower their blood pressure.[44] Krill oil is particularly helpful for people with arthritis. Arthritis is an inflammatory condition of the joints, and you know by now that omega-3s have potent anti-inflammatory effects. Think of omega-3s as lubricant for stiff, swollen, painful joints, making them function more smoothly. A double-blind placebo-controlled trial showed that among people with cardiovascular disease and/ or rheumatoid arthritis or osteoarthritis, who also had elevated levels of the inflammatory marker C-reactive protein, 300 mg of krill oil daily for three weeks reduced their levels of C-reactive protein by about 32 percent, while CRP actually *increased* by as much as 32 percent in the placebo group. The krill-oil group also had significantly reduced pain, stiffness, and functional impairment.[45]

How about PMS? In a double-blind randomized trial testing 70 patients with PMS, with half taking fish oil and half taking krill oil, those on krill oil showed significantly improved dysmenorrhea (painful periods) as well as the emotional symptoms associated with PMS. Women taking krill oil needed fewer pain-relieving medications than those taking fish oil. Another study reinforced that krill oil is more effective than fish oil for improving not only the emotional symptoms of PMS but also breast tenderness and joint pain. The study authors noted that these benefits may have been due to the omega-3s counteracting, or at least lessening, the inflammation that was driven by inflammatory compounds derived from omega-6 fats.[46] So if you're a woman of reproductive age and you experience difficult and painful periods, omega-3 supplementation (particularly with krill oil) might help, but also be sure to cut back on omega-6 in your diet.

As a maintenance dose—if you're already healthy and want to stay that way—we recommend 500 mg daily of krill oil. As a therapeutic dose—if you're addressing a condition that may respond to increased omega-3s—we recommend 1 to 3 grams.

Gamma Linolenic Acid (GLA)

We've spent a significant portion of this book warning you about the dangers of consuming too much omega-6, which comes mostly in the form of industrial seed oils used in processed foods and cooking oils. But we also mentioned that linoleic acid, the parent omega-6, is, in fact, an "essential" fatty acid. You do need *some.* More importantly, you need the conversion processes that turn linoleic acid into its downstream products to be functioning optimally. Your body doesn't waste precious energy doing things for no reason. If it's going to the effort of converting linoleic acid into other things, then you definitely need those other things, too. Even the pro-inflammatory molecules that come from the omega-6 pathway are necessary; they're a problem only when you consume excess quantities.

One of the compounds produced in the omega-6 conversion pathway is gamma linolenic acid (GLA). GLA is itself converted into another kind of fat, called DGLA (dihomo-gamma-linolenic acid). Both GLA and DGLA are mainly found in your cell membranes, rather than being freely available in your body. Remember what we said about those cell membranes: if they don't work right, *you* don't work right. In supplement form, GLA is found in borage oil (20 to 27 percent GLA), black currant seed oil (15 to 20 percent GLA), evening primrose oil (7 to 14 percent GLA), or hemp-seed oil (1.7 percent GLA). If delta-6-desaturase (D6D), the first enzyme in the conversion pathway, is not working properly, you might need to get GLA directly from one of these supplements because your body won't produce much of it. What interferes with D6D? The top culprits include advanced age, alcohol abuse, smoking, insulin resistance, consumption of trans fats and partially hydrogenated oils, or insufficient zinc, magnesium, vitamins C, E, B6, or B3.[47]

As we've discussed, omega-3 fats are usually building blocks for anti-inflammatory compounds, and omega-6 fats are usually building blocks for compounds that are pro-inflammatory. But that's not always the case; *some* omega-6 fats can result in beneficial anti-inflammatory signals, and DGLA is one of them. DGLA is believed to help facilitate blood-vessel dilation and protect against dangerous blood clotting, just like you would expect from an omega-3.[48]

Further evidence of GLA as an *anti*-inflammatory omega-6 fat comes from studies in patients with rheumatoid arthritis (RA). One study showed that supplementing with GLA from borage oil (1.4 grams daily for 6 months) significantly improved joint tenderness, swelling, and pain; while cottonseed oil, a high-omega-6 oil used as a placebo, showed no benefit.[49] Similar benefits were found in another study in RA patients given 2.8 grams of GLA a day for 12 months, with 16 of 21 patients showing meaningful improvement,[50] and compared to soybean oil, 6 months of supplementing daily with 2 grams of GLA from black currant seed oil improved joint tenderness in 34 patients with RA.[51,52]

GLA may be especially good for skin health, which is why some cosmetic products—especially ones claiming to restore radiance and glow to your skin—contain borage, evening primrose, or black currant seed oils. Patients with atopic dermatitis have been noted to have a reduced conversion of linoleic acid to GLA,[53] and evening primrose oil has been shown to benefit patients with atopic dermatitis or eczema.[54] Infants, particularly ones who are not breastfed, may benefit from GLA or DGLA supplementation. Breast milk contains these special fats, but commercial formulas don't, and D6D activity is thought to be insufficient during this early stage of life, which would deprive formula-fed infants of these fats.[55] Symptoms of GLA/DGLA deficiency include dry, thick skin, skin eruptions resembling eczema, and growth failure.[56]

The anti-inflammatory effects of GLA have been observed in other health conditions. Supplementing with GLA plus EPA was shown to benefit patients with mild-to-moderate asthma, decreasing reliance on rescue medications and improving subjective quality of life.[57] Women with premenstrual syndrome (PMS) have been noted to have an impaired conversion of linoleic acid to GLA, and evening primrose oil may help women with PMS.[58]

Evening primrose oil was also shown to benefit ADHD patients with low zinc levels. Low-zinc status impairs the conversion of linoleic acid to GLA; researchers speculated that the supplemental GLA may have compensated for the low zinc.[59]

Disease States That May Benefit from GLA Supplementation (with or without EPA/DHA)

- Atopic dermatitis; eczema
- Premenstrual syndrome (PMS)
- Autoimmune disease (especially rheumatoid arthritis)
- ADHD
- Osteoporosis[60]
- Dry eye syndrome[61]

Argan Oil

Argan oil is almost exclusively produced in southwestern Morocco, where the argan tree grows.[62] It has been used in Morocco for centuries as an edible and topical oil. The Amazigh, who are natives of the Argan forests, traditionally extracted edible argan oil from the kernels of the argan fruit stones, and this oil is a staple in the Amazigh diet.[63] Argan oil has been noted for improving many skin ailments, such as acne, psoriasis, eczema, dry skin, and wrinkles, and it may even help to prevent hair loss and improve dry hair.[64] For these reasons, like GLA-rich borage, evening primrose, and black currant seed oils, you'll see argan oil listed among the ingredients on cosmetics for skin and hair care.

Today, edible virgin argan oil is typically extracted from slightly roasted kernels, which may denature the oil.[65,66] The fruit kernel of the argan tree provides the oil, which is copper in color and has a flavor similar to hazelnuts. Virgin argan oil used in beauty products comes from unroasted kernels, and it's golden in color and virtually tasteless. However, it is less stable than edible virgin argan oil.

Argan oil is rich in tocopherols, which are compounds with vitamin E activity and antioxidant properties. The tocopherol content is thought to contribute to some of argan oil's health benefits.[67] There are a few different forms of tocopherol. Many vitamin E supplements contain only alpha-tocopherol, but it's gamma-tocopherol that's believed to be one of the best free-radical scavengers, and this potent antioxidant makes up 69 percent of the total tocopherols in argan oil.[68] Olive oil contains some tocopherols as well—women have used olive oil topically for their skin and hair for centuries—but argan oil contains nearly twice the tocopherol concentration of olive oil.

The argan oil used in cosmetic products is thought to have moisturizing and wound-healing properties, as well as anti-aging, anti-acne, and antisebum (oil) effects. One study found that four weeks of twice-daily application of a cream containing argan oil plus extracts from sesame and saw palmetto reduced greasiness and improved the appearance of oily facial skin.[69] The study was small—only 20 subjects—but it included men and women, and almost all of them reported a noticeable improvement in facial-skin oiliness, so this isn't exclusively the purview of women looking to boost their beauty routine. It probably sounds strange to apply oil, or a product containing oil, to your face if it's already oily. But there's a method behind the madness: it may not be simply that your skin is producing too much oil; it may be that too much is being secreted because of an imbalance in the fats in your skin. Correct the balance, correct the problem.

Argan oil contains less than 0.5 percent omega-3, yet it imparts some of the cardiovascular benefits typically observed with omega-3 supplementation. In rats, argan oil has been shown to reduce total cholesterol, triglycerides, and LDL,[70] although it's up for debate whether that last one matters much for heart health. In humans, argan oil was shown to lower triglycerides and raise HDL,[71] and this ratio—lower triglycerides and higher HDL—is a strong indicator of cardiometabolic health. Other protective compounds in argan oil help protect LDL particles against oxidation,[72] and as noted earlier, LDL particles per se aren't heart-health enemy number one, but *oxidized* LDL can cause trouble.

Other studies corroborate a beneficial effect for argan oil on cardiovascular status.[73] In type 2 diabetics with abnormal blood lipids, taking 25 milliliters of argan oil daily (a little more than 1.5 tablespoons) for just three weeks reduced triglycerides, total cholesterol, LDL, and oxidation of LDL, while increasing HDL.[74] A control group consuming butter experienced none of these changes. When it comes to markers for cardiovascular health, little-known argan oil seems to be a jack of all trades, to the point where researchers went so far as to say that argan oil can "be recommended in the nutritional management of type 2 diabetes."[75] Considering that cardiovascular problems are the number one killer of people with type 2 diabetes, this is no small feat.

In people with unhealthy cholesterol levels, taking 25 milliliters per day of edible virgin argan oil at breakfast for three weeks reduced platelet aggregation and increased HDL by an impressive 26 percent.[76] Similar to the study mentioned above, these benefits were not found with butter. In both animal and human studies, argan oil has been found to inhibit platelet aggregation and reduce oxidative stress.[77,78] Studies in rats show that argan oil has the potential to improve blood pressure, blood glucose levels, and insulin resistance,[79] and also improve blood-vessel function, blood pressure, and blood-glucose levels in hypertensive or diabetic rats.[80,81,82]

Here again, we see argan oil mimicking the effects of omega-3s, even though argan oil is actually high in omega-6. You can see now why we're so infuriated by alarmist headlines about fats and oils. Things are rarely as simple as they're made out to be in the news.

The proposed therapeutic dosage of argan oil to help with cardiometabolic disease is 1 to 2 tablespoons (15 to 30 milliliters) of edible uncooked virgin argan oil per day, with a dose more suited for maintenance of good health as just ½ to 1 teaspoon per day (3 to 6 milliliters). Argan oil can be used on salads and may be used for cooking, but owing to the high omega-6 content, we caution against cooking at high temperatures.[83]

Healthy Oil Supplement Recommendations

- **Fish or Algal oil:** 3 to 4 grams per day (combined EPA and DHA) for maintenance of good health; more may be warranted for those with inflammatory or cardiometabolic disease

- **Krill oil:** 500 mg daily as a maintenance dose; 1 to 3 grams daily for those dealing with a condition that may respond to increased omega-3s

- **Alpha-linolenic acid:** 2.5 to 5 grams per day to maintain good health; 5 to 10 grams daily from flaxseed or ALA-enriched foods in order to reduce inflammation

- **GLA:** 400 to 3,000 mg daily for conditions that may respond to extra GLA (especially skin issues and PMS); supplementation is not necessary for everyday health maintenance

- **Argan oil:** ½ to 1 teaspoon (3 to 6 milliliters) daily for maintenance of good health; 1 to 2 tablespoons (15 to 30 milliliters) of uncooked virgin argan oil daily for those with cardiometabolic disease

Summary

- There's more to all of this than "omega-3s are good and omega-6s are bad." Both linoleic acid (LA) and alpha-linoleic acid (ALA) convert into highly valuable, inflammation-reducing fats.

- Medium-chain triglycerides (MCTs), such as coconut oil, are saturated fats that are 6 to 12 carbons in length. They are particularly good for burning fat.

- While we recommend eating whole foods as often as possible, sometimes it is necessary to supplement.

- Fish oil: Make sure your fish oil is not overly processed, and that it contains high levels of DHA as well as EPA.

- Krill oil is like fish oil, only better: it is less likely to contain mercury or other contaminants, and it provides you with your long-chain omega-3s in a form that is easily absorbed and used by the body.

- GLA, a downstream benefit of LA, can reduce inflammation, and has been shown to help with rheumatoid arthritis, PMS, ADHD, and other conditions. It can be found in borage oil, evening primrose oil, and black currant seed oil, and these are fine to take in supplement form.

- Argan oil is particularly good for the skin and for cardiovascular health, and it can be used topically or as a supplement; it should not be used for cooking.

CHAPTER 9

WHAT TO EAT: THE RIGHT FOODS FOR THE RIGHT FATS

Targeted supplementation with the fats and oils that are appropriate for you can help you restore and maintain a healthy balance of fats in your body, priming your cells and your mitochondria for optimal health. But supplements are just that—supplemental to a nutritious diet based on whole, unprocessed foods. In this chapter, we'll walk you through which foods to eat and which foods to avoid to help you reach a healthy balance of fats. As you'll remember from early in the book, we, along with the U.S. National Institutes of Health (NIH), recommend 650 mg of EPA and DHA, 2.22 grams of ALA, and 4.44 grams of LA for adults daily.[1] This equates to an omega-6-to-3 ratio of about 2:1.

AQUATIC SOURCES OF DIETARY FAT

In Tables 9.1 and 9.2, we present the omega-3 content of select seafood items you're likely to find at your local supermarket, as well as their omega-3-to-6 ratios. If you live in an area with a good fishmonger, or someone in your life enjoys fishing, you may have access to a wider variety of fish and shellfish.

Table 9.1: Dietary Sources of Marine Omega-3s[2,3]

Dietary Source	EPA/DHA omega-3s (grams per/ 3 oz. serving)
Salmon roe	2.70
Halibut	2.21
Herring	1.7–1.8
Salmon (wild)	1.0–3.0
Sardines	1.0–1.74
Trout	1.0
Oysters	0.45–1.15
Mackerel	0.35–1.80
Tuna (fresh)	0.25–1.30

Table 9.2: Long-Chain Omega-3-to-6 Ratio of Select Seafood[4]

Dietary Source	Omega-3-to-6 Ratio
Sardines	16.5
Halibut	14
Cod	13.4
Anglerfish	9.3
Mackerel	8.4
Tuna	5.8
Salmon (wild)	5.5

Don't Ruin a Good Thing

While aquatic animals and plants have been our traditional sources for DHA/EPA omega-3 fats, the presence of environmental pollutants such as mercury, lead, dioxins, and other contaminants is an important issue if you're looking to achieve and maintain optimal health. Moreover, modern food-production techniques mean that more fish are bred in aquatic farms, where they're fed pellets made from grain that is typically GMO and/or sprayed with glyphosate, rather than consuming their natural diet of marine plants and smaller prey fish and other aquatic life. When fish consume less natural omega-3s, their fat contains less omega-3s, so it's best to choose wild-caught fish from clean waters whenever possible.

As if that weren't enough, the grain pellets used as feed may contain antibiotics, and drugs and other toxic chemicals may also be used in farm-raised seafood due to the buildup of bacteria and fecal matter in the overfilled ponds.[5] There may even be growth hormones added to farm-raised shrimp, as opposed to organic shrimp.[6] The nonprofit organization Public Citizen wrote, "Considered as a whole, the presence of antibiotics such as chloramphenicol, toxic chemical compounds that include persistent organic pollutants (POPs), and pesticides used to farm raise aquatic species, demand that consumers require further investigation by scientists and health authorities into the health risks of farmed-raised shrimp."[7]

If you read Larry Olmstead's excellent book *Real Food/Fake Food*, you will realize that shrimp is the single most consumed seafood in the United States. We eat more pounds of shrimp than any other fish. Up to 90 percent of the shrimp consumed in the U.S. is imported from other countries, but it appears that less than 2 percent is inspected by U.S. regulatory agencies. Nevertheless, in 2015, the FDA had a record number of import refusals for shrimp. This happens when shrimp is tested and found to contain unacceptable contaminants, such as banned antibiotics or elevated levels of toxins. Some of the antibiotics used in shrimp farming are not allowed in American food production because they've been deemed carcinogenic. Olmsted recommends avoiding shrimp in restaurants unless you're absolutely convinced the shrimp were indeed caught in the Gulf of Mexico.

Canned salmon, sardines, mackerel, and other fish are convenient and economical ways to consume more seafood, but try to avoid making canned seafood the primary source of omega-3 in your diet. High heat is often used during the canning process, which may oxidize the fragile fats. Stick to organic canned seafood, and if you like to dress up canned seafood with mayonnaise, use an organic mayonnaise and opt for one made from avocado oil, rather than soybean oil, in order to minimize the omega-6. It is also best to avoid sardines in olive oil and get the ones in water, as the olive oil used in canned sardines is inferior and not at all high quality.

Additionally, be mindful of how you cook your seafood. Knowing what you know now about the dangers of vegetable and seed oils, you definitely don't want to fry fish in those oils. Poach, steam, or bake fish instead of frying so you don't add damaged, oxidized omega-6 to an otherwise nutritious meal. Baked fish is associated with health benefits,[8] but fried fish is not. This is most likely because of the cooking oils typically used for frying.

If you're a ceviche, sushi, or sashimi lover, you might be best off of all. Raw preparations made with wild-caught seafood from safe, clean sources is one of the best ways to get marine omega-3s, because when kept raw, you can be certain none of the fragile fats have been damaged. Fish or salmon roe are probably the highest density of healthy EPA/DHA that you can get, in addition to being loaded with phosphatidylcholine.

WHOLE NUTS AND SEEDS

Consuming whole, intact nuts and seeds is a world apart from consuming industrial seed oils. Just like the oils extracted from them, nuts and seeds are high in omega-6, but when you consume them in their intact form, they're naturally packaged with antioxidants that help protect against oxidation, not to mention also coming along with fiber, vitamins, and minerals, which the extracted oils don't deliver. Since heat is one of the factors that damages fragile omega-6 and omega-3 fats, your best bet might be to consume raw nuts and seeds, if your stomach can handle it.

In Table 9.3 we've provided the breakdown of saturated, mono-unsaturated, and polyunsaturated fats in commonly consumed nuts and seeds, along with their omega-6-to-3 ratios. While some of them, such as peanuts (not a nut but a legume), Brazil nuts, and almonds, appear to have extremely high omega-6-to-3 ratios, keep in mind that polyunsaturated fat makes up less than half of their total fat, and it's closer to only a third or less. Those nuts are higher in monounsaturated fat than polyunsaturated, so even though their omega-6-to-3 ratios are very high, the total amount of omega-6 you would get from them is less than what you'd get from consuming the same amount of sunflower seeds or pecans, which are higher in total omega-6 even though their ratios are lower.

Table 9.3: Fatty Acid Composition of Commonly Consumed Nuts and Seeds[9] (grams per 1-ounce serving)

Nut or seed	SFA	MUFA	PUFA	% PUFA	Total Omega-6	Total Omega-3	Omega-6-to-3 Ratio
Flaxseeds	1.0	2.1	8.0	72%	1.7	6.4	0.27
Chia seeds	0.9	0.6	6.5	81%	1.6	4.9	0.33
Walnuts	1.7	2.5	13.3	76%	10.8	2.6	4.2
Macadamias	3.4	16.6	0.4	2%	0.37	.058	6.4
Pecans	1.7	11.5	6.1	32%	5.8	0.28	20.7
Pistachios	1.5	6.5	3.8	32%	3.7	0.072	51.4
Sesame seeds	1.9	5.3	6.1	46%	6.0	0.10	60.0
Hazelnuts	1.3	12.8	2.2	13%	2.2	0.025	88.0
Pumpkin seeds (pepitas)	2.5	4.0	5.9	48%	5.8	0.051	113.7
Pine nuts (pignolis)	1.4	5.3	9.6	59%	9.5	0.032	297.0

Nut or seed	SFA	MUFA	PUFA	% PUFA	Total Omega-6	Total Omega-3	Omega-6-to-3 Ratio
Sunflower seeds	1.2	5.2	6.5	50%	6.5	0.021	309.5
Brazil nuts	4.3	6.9	5.8	34%	5.8	0.005	1160.0
Almonds	1.0	8.6	3.4	26%	3.4	0.002	1700.0
Peanuts	1.9	6.8	4.4	34%	4.4	0.0008	5500.0

COMMON OILS

Some oils are better than others! Table 9.4 shows the omega-6-to-3 ratios of common oils, but please note that this isn't the whole story. Olive oil and coconut oil, for example, have properties that are great for you besides just their 6:3 status, and flaxseed oil is better for you than canola oil, even though canola oil has the best 6:3 ratio on this chart. This table offers a range of oils high in ALA. Table 9.5 in turn offers some good dietary sources of ALA.

Table 9.4: The Omega-6-to-3 Ratio* of Common Oils[10,11]

Dietary Source	Omega-6-to-3 ratio
Grapeseed	696
Sesame	138
Safflower	78
Sunflower	68
Cottonseed	54
Corn	46
Peanut	32
Olive	13
Avocado	13
Soybean	7
Hemp seeds	3
Chia seeds	0.33
Flaxseeds	0.27
Canola	0.2

*The omega-6:3 ratio here refers to LA/ALA.

Table 9.5: Good Dietary Sources of ALA: From Highest to Lowest[12]

Dietary Source	Grams of ALA per Tablespoon (15 ml/12.35 grams)
Walnuts (English)	2.6
Flaxseeds	2.4–2.8
Chia seeds	2.1
Soybeans	1.6
Walnut oil, oats (germ)	1.4
Canola oil	1.3
Soybean oil	1.23
Seaweed	0.80
Wheat (germ)	0.70
Beans	0.60
Eggs	0.10–0.60
Almonds, purslane	0.40
Rice (bran)	0.20
Walnuts (black)	0.16
Olive oil	0.10

THE BENEFITS OF FLAXSEED

The long-chain marine omega-3 fats EPA and DHA are the most potent for inducing the beneficial cardiometabolic effects that omega-3s are known for. But remember that the parent omega-3, alpha-linolenic acid (ALA) also has plenty to offer. Consuming flaxseeds has consistently been found to reduce inflammation and platelet aggregation (clotting).[13,14,15,16,17] In people with elevated cholesterol, ALA has been shown to decrease C-reactive protein, that key marker of inflammation. Researchers attribute the reduction in inflammation seen from consuming more ALA to increases in EPA and DPA in the blood through conversion. Now as we've discussed, most people don't make that conversion very effectively, but this goes to show that if you supplement with ALA, you'll still end up with some DHA and EPA.[18]

In a different study, obese subjects given 30 grams of flaxseed meal a day (providing 5 grams of ALA) for two weeks had significant reductions in inflammation compared to those given a placebo.[19] Flaxseed meal has been shown to reduce triglycerides and improve the ratio of total cholesterol to HDL in patients with elevated cholesterol.[20] Flaxseeds have shown beneficial effects in clinical studies on other risk factors associated with cardiovascular disease: they improve insulin sensitivity,[21] lower triglyceride levels,[22] and reduce small-dense LDL particles.[23] They've also been shown to protect against some of the harmful effects of consuming a high amount of trans fats.[24] Not bad for something you can grind fresh and sprinkle on yogurt or cottage cheese or put into a smoothie.

Just like fish oil, flaxseeds are polyunsaturated and thus highly susceptible to oxidation and rancidity. It's best to purchase whole flaxseeds and grind them fresh right before consuming. (A coffee grinder or spice grinder is the perfect tool for this.) Store your seeds or any unused grounds away from heat and light—refrigeration is ideal. You can also soak the flaxseeds overnight and put them in your smoothie in the morning. We do not recommend the use of flax oil, as it is processed, and therefore highly susceptible to oxidative damage and going rancid.

In case you're curious, brown flaxseeds have slightly more ALA than golden flaxseeds do, but the difference is fairly minor, so use whichever you prefer. They both have a very pleasant nutty flavor. Flaxseeds are an extremely rich source of ALA, but if you don't like flax, you can get ALA from eggs that come from hens whose feed includes flaxseeds. ALA-enriched eggs have five times more ALA than conventional eggs.[25] Walnuts also contain ALA, but they're far higher in total omega-6 than omega-3, so don't rely on walnuts as your main source of ALA.

Potential benefits of flaxseed:

- Decreased blood pressure
- Decreased inflammation
- Decreased blood clotting
- Reduced atherosclerosis
- Decreased small-dense LDL, triglycerides, and total cholesterol/HDL ratio

Dose of ALA to reduce inflammation:

- 5 to 10 grams per day from flaxseed or ALA-enriched foods

THE GRASS-FED DIFFERENCE

As we've mentioned throughout this book, seafood isn't the only source of DHA/EPA. It's the most concentrated source, so consuming seafood is a convenient way to get a substantial amount of these crucial fats; but if you're allergic to fish or shellfish, or you simply don't enjoy the flavor, you can get ALA but very little EPA and DHA from land-based animals. Meat from grain-fed cattle contains a small amount of omega-3, but meat from grass-fed animals will give you more (particularly the omega-3 ALA).

According to researchers who've studied the differences in the fat composition of meat from grass-fed and grain-fed cattle, when grain is added to a grass diet, the concentration of omega-3s in the meat decreases. Not only does it decrease, but the relationship is linear: the more grain a steer consumes, the lower the omega-3 in its meat.[26] Compared to meat from grain-fed animals, meat from grass-fed animals consistently contains from 2 to 11 times more ALA, 2 to 5 times more EPA, and approximately twice as much DHA.

Moreover, the higher amount of omega-3 in grass-fed animals comes without any significant increase in omega-6, so meat from grass-fed cattle has a more favorable omega-6-to-3 ratio.[27] In meat from grass-fed animals, the omega-6-to-3 ratio is an ideal 2:1. Compare that to meat from grain-fed animals, where the ratio can be as high as 13:1!

Most of the lamb, goat, and bison produced in the U.S. are still raised on pasture, so looking specifically for grass-fed meats is more important when you're selecting beef. Your best bet for finding meat that was grass-fed and grass-*finished* is to find a farmer in your area raising his or her animals on pasture, but grass-fed meats are increasingly available in supermarkets across the U.S. The American Grassfed Association is the best certification out there to confirm compliance with these standards, so look for their seal.

Conjugated Linoleic Acid (CLA)

Apart from the increased omega-3 content, grass-fed beef provides another distinct advantage over grain-fed beef in the form of special fats collectively called CLA. CLA, short for conjugated linoleic acid, is a trans fat, but unlike the harmful trans fats produced from the partial hydrogenation of vegetable and seed oils, this naturally occurring trans fat has been shown to be beneficial for health.

CLA improves blood lipids and insulin sensitivity, stimulates bone mineralization, and also has anticlotting, anti-atherosclerotic, and anticancer effects.[28,29] Researchers have written, "Over the past two decades numerous studies have shown significant health benefits attributable to the actions of CLA, as demonstrated by experimental animal models, including actions to reduce carcinogenesis, atherosclerosis, and onset of diabetes. Conjugated linoleic acid has also been reported to modulate body composition by reducing the accumulation of adipose tissue in a variety of species including mice, rats, pigs, and now humans."[30] Perhaps the near disappearance of CLA from the modern Western diet is a contributing factor to the obesity epidemic and the explosion in chronic diseases during the past several decades.

CLA is produced via bacterial fermentation in the digestive tract of ruminant animals such as cows, goats, sheep, and bison, and it becomes concentrated in the meat and dairy products produced from these animals. Pigs, chickens, and turkeys may also contain small amounts of CLA. In the era of industrial feedlots, beef and dairy cattle have been removed from the grassy pastures that would have them producing far more CLA in their meat and milk than animals consuming most of their feed as grain. More CLA is another reason besides increased omega-3s to favor meat and dairy from grass-fed animals. And the good news is that you don't have to eat meat to get your CLA: you can easily get it from pastured butter—milk from grass-fed cows contains as much as *500 percent more CLA* than milk from grain-fed cows.[31]

The total amount of CLA even in grass-fed meat is low: beef fat contains just 1.7 to 10.8 mg of CLA per gram of fat,[32] but don't dismiss the importance of even just this small amount. Remember what we said about vitamins and minerals: these are compounds your body needs in only miniscule amounts, but the consequences of not getting those tiny amounts can be devastating.

Evidence supports a beneficial role for CLA in reducing body fat and supporting the maintenance of lean muscle tissue,[33] because remember, if you're trying to lose weight, you want to lose *fat*, not muscle or other lean tissue. Studies show that this can be achieved even in the absence of alterations in diet and physical activity levels,[34] meaning that CLA may help you lose fat even without changing your diet or exercise habits. We weren't kidding when we said fats send important signals to your cells!

CLA has been shown to reduce the synthesis of new body fat and to increase your body's capacity to burn fat. As we've discussed, fats are burned—converted to energy—in your mitochondria. There's an enzyme called carnitine palmitoyl-transferase-1 (CPT-1) that helps transport fats into your mitochondria, and CLA increases the activity of this enzyme while *decreasing* activity of enzymes involved in telling your body to generate and store fat.[35]

Optimal dietary intake of CLA has been estimated to be as low as 95 mg per day and as high as 3,000 mg per day. Considering that most Americans consume only around 150 to 200 mg of CLA a day, you're likely near the low end of the range, especially if you don't regularly consume meat or dairy products from grass-fed animals. We recommend 500 to 1,000 mg of CLA daily, which is closer to the amount humans likely consumed during Paleolithic times.[36]

Grass-Fed Beef: Benefits beyond the Fats

Moving beyond fats, it might surprise you to learn that beef is a rich source of vitamins and minerals. You're probably accustomed to automatically picturing brightly colored fruits and vegetables when you think about these essential nutrients, but beef is loaded with B vitamins, iron, zinc, selenium, and more.

If you've ever bought grass-fed beef, you might have noticed the fat has a distinct yellow appearance. This is due to its beta-carotene content—that's right, the same beta-carotene responsible for the orange pigments in carrots and sweet potatoes shows itself in the fat of grass-fed animals. Green grasses contain beta-carotene, and because cattle consume grass in such large quantities, the pigment becomes concentrated in their fat.[37] You'll also notice a stark difference in color if you compare butter from exclusively grass-fed dairy cows and that from grain-fed animals. Be sure to read labels though, because some manufacturers add synthetic coloring to their butter and especially to margarine and other vegetable oil spreads specifically for the purpose of mimicking the color of authentic butter from grass-fed cows. Don't let them deceive you. Buy the real thing.

Meat from grass-fed animals contains as much as seven times more beta-carotene than meat from grain-fed animals. Beta-carotene is a precursor to vitamin A, which is critical for your eye health and visual acuity, bone health, reproductive function, respiratory system, and more. Vitamin A is required for the production and function of white blood cells, and it helps maintain the integrity of your skin as well as that of your small intestine. These are among your body's first-line defenses against toxins and pathogenic organisms, so having enough beta-carotene and vitamin A may contribute to a robust immune system. (In your grandparents' day, everyone took a spoonful of vitamin A–rich cod liver oil daily in order to ward off colds and other illnesses.) Buy meat, cheese, yogurt, and other dairy products sourced from grass-fed animals whenever possible.

Another nutrient available from beef is vitamin E, and grass-fed meat contains between two and ten times as much vitamin E as grain-fed meat.[38] Vitamin E is a key antioxidant that may help to prevent oxidation of the beef fat itself, and also may contribute to your body's antioxidant pool to protect against oxidative damage to the fats in your body.

Have you ever noticed that if meat sits around for a little while, it changes color? Fresh beef is a bright, vibrant red, but beef that's not as fresh—like you might see marked down for quick sale at the store—looks brown. We recommend avoiding beef that has turned brown, as this indicates oxidative deterioration of one of the proteins that contributes to the red color. Grass-fed meat retains its bright red color longer than grain-fed meat, which may be due to its higher vitamin E content lending protection against oxidation.[39]

Meat from grass-fed animals contains other important antioxidants as well. Remember glutathione, "the master antioxidant"? It's found in every cell in your body, and it's a primary player in how your liver neutralizes toxic compounds. Beyond its role in detoxification, glutathione is a powerful scavenger of the free radicals that cause oxidative damage to your DNA and the structural fats and other components of your tissues. Meat and vegetables contain high amounts of glutathione, and since lush green forages are high in glutathione, meat from animals raised on pasture is higher in glutathione than that from grain-fed animals.[40]

Grass-fed meats are also higher in two other free radical–neutralizing antioxidants, called superoxide dismutase and catalase.[41] Just like with vitamin E, the higher concentration of antioxidant enzymes in grass-fed meat helps to protect the fats in the meat from oxidizing during exposure to air as well as during cooking. So just as grass-fed meat is richer in fragile omega-3 fats, it also contains higher levels of antioxidants that help protect these fats.[42]

The benefits of grass-fed over grain-fed meat:

- Higher concentration of omega-3 in the form of ALA
- Lower concentration of omega-6
- Lower omega-6-to-3 ratio
- Higher concentration of trans-vaccenic acid
- Higher concentration of CLA
- Higher in precursors for vitamins A and E
- Higher in antioxidants such as glutathione, superoxide dismutase, and catalase
- Lower amounts of trans-oleic (10t-18:1) fat
- Less fat oxidation

PUTTING IT ALL TOGETHER: TIPS TO STAY HEALTHY

Consume Seafood

By far the most efficient and effective way to increase your consumption of omega-3s, particularly EPA and DHA, is to eat more food from the sea. Whenever possible, purchase wild-caught seafood harvested from clean waters and limit your consumption of farm-raised seafood, as it's likely higher in harmful contaminants.[43] As mentioned earlier, compared to wild-caught fish, farmed fish contains less omega-3 and more omega-6 due to the feed they're given. (Be aware that some farmed salmon use healthy marine feed, and if you decide to buy farmed salmon, look for quality farmed salmon with a documented level of EPA and DHA that has not been given any antibiotics.)[44] Less of the good stuff and more of the bad stuff—not the way you want to go for your health.

Consume Foods from Pastured Animals

Choose meat, butter, cheese, eggs, milk, and other foods from animals raised on organic pastures. This will give you more of the crucial omega-3s and CLA while also providing more beta-carotene and other vitamins and minerals.[45,46] Inquire with local farmers in your area about their animal-husbandry practices. Many small farms raise animals humanely on pastures free from pesticides and genetically modified grasses, but they're not certified organic. The paperwork required to obtain organic certification may be prohibitively burdensome for a small family farm even though their practices are in line with—or even better than—official organic standards.

For other ways to get omega-3 fats, consider purchasing eggs from hens raised on pasture. They provide as much as ten times more omega-3 than conventional eggs, and they're also higher in vitamins D, B12, and folic acid.[47] But remember: all these nutrients are in the yolks, so don't be afraid to enjoy whole eggs. No more egg-white omelets!

Cook meat and eggs at a low-to-medium temperature to ensure you minimize the oxidation of the fats and cholesterol in these foods. While we generally recommend against reheating in a microwave, simply because it increases the chance of oxidation, we understand that leftovers are an important part of anyone's diet. Just be sure to use a low-power setting (50 percent power or less) to heat foods and beverages that contain fat and cholesterol.

Regarding other animal foods, the linoleic acid content of chicken fat is 13.5 percent,[48] while pork is 8 percent,[49] compared to just 2.7 percent for beef.[50] Pork fat is predominantly saturated and monounsaturated, so the total amount of polyunsaturated fat is low, but of that amount, there's far more omega-6 than omega-3. The same goes for chicken: chicken fat is mostly monounsaturated, but it has a substantial amount of polyunsaturated fat, and that portion is high in omega-6.

Of course, free-range chickens that have access to green grasses as well as grubs and worms (in addition to organic grain) have a better nutrient profile than chickens raised in massive indoor confinement operations and fed genetically modified grains. Pigs allowed to forage in wooded areas may have an improved nutrient profile compared to feedlot pigs. Choose organic non-CAFO (Concentrated Animal Feeding Operation) chicken and pork whenever possible, or buy lean meats and add olive oil or avocado oil for flavor.

Consume Nuts and Seeds in Moderation

Choose organic nuts and seeds, and if you prefer roasted instead of raw, purchase nuts and seeds that have been roasted without any industrial seed oils. (Many popular brands of nuts are roasted with soybean or cottonseed oils.) If you enjoy flavored or seasoned varieties, avoid honey-roasted nuts, which are typically made with sugar and corn syrup. Read labels and stick with versions where you can pronounce and understand the ingredients: cumin, cayenne, turmeric, or cocoa powder, for example. If you have insulin resistance or a related cardio-metabolic issue, we advise limiting consumption of high-omega-6 nuts and seeds such as walnuts, pine nuts, sunflower and pumpkin seeds, as these may contribute to higher insulin levels.

Add Flaxseed to Your Food

Avoid consuming flax oil, which is highly susceptible to oxidation and does not appear to provide the same health benefits as freshly ground flaxseeds. Instead, we suggest adding 1 to 3 tablespoons of flaxseed to your diet, either by soaking them overnight or by grinding them fresh. This is particularly necessary if your intake of ALA from other sources, such as leafy greens, is low. Freshly ground flax can be added to yogurt, cottage cheese, smoothies, or oatmeal for a convenient omega-3 boost.

Avoid Trans Fats and Industrial Seed Oils

Industrial seed oils are hidden in almost all processed foods, from baked goods to condiments, and even in places where you'd never expect them to be lurking, such as in bread crumbs. Foods typically high in trans fats and seed oils include salad dressings, cake frostings, mayonnaise, fried foods, margarine and vegetable shortening, pastries, peanut butter, crackers, and processed snacks such as potato chips. Read labels; you'll be stunned at the unexpected places these oils pop up.

﹀

You've probably gathered by now that the *Superfuel* way of eating is a little different from how you might be accustomed to thinking about food. You might find yourself spending a bit more time cooking than calling for takeout or picking something up from the prepared hot foods bar at the supermarket. You may also spend a little more time at the store, reading labels and looking for those sneaky seed oils. Pretty soon though, choosing the right foods will be second nature and you won't even need to think about it. It won't be long before you're an expert and your shopping and food preparation will be as quick and easy as they've always been. Your health is worth it. It's a small investment of time and effort that will pay enormous dividends for your long-term health and quality of life.

CONCLUSION

Now that you understand the power of the ratio of omega-6 to omega-3 fats in your diet, and the vital role this plays in your physical, mental, and cognitive health, it's time to move past outdated government guidelines that encourage consumption of large amounts of industrial seed oils. If you've followed recommendations to eat a high-carbohydrate, low-fat diet, and you've dutifully avoided animal fats in favor of the "vegetable" oils you were led to believe were good for you, yet you've struggled to lose weight or get healthy, it's time to leave those old, *failed* recommendations where they belong: in the dustbin of history.

When implementing our recommended cyclical ketogenic diet while you're shopping, target foods high in healthy omega-3 fats, avoid high-carbohydrate foods, and remember that your health begins at the cellular level. You're only as healthy as your cells—and their membranes. Your cells make up your organs, glands, muscles, and other tissues. All those cells need healthy fats. Superfuel your body with healthy fats that come from whole, unprocessed foods. Foods that were grown or raised without adulteration or chemical manipulation and without harmful additives, which take away from their life-sustaining properties: organically grown vegetables, fruits, nuts and seeds, beef, pork, chicken, eggs, dairy, and other foods from animals raised on species-appropriate diets in healthy environments; and wild-caught seafood from clean, sustainable sources.

You are not only what *you* eat, but you're also what you eat *ate*. Consuming food that comes from healthy animals that are allowed to forage and graze outdoors in fresh air, sunlight, and green pastures that are uncontaminated with herbicides, and do not feed on GMO grains loaded with omega-6, will give you the most bang for your nutritional buck. Not only does this affect the concentration and quality of the nutrients and especially the fats in those foods, but in turn, it affects the nutrients and fats in *you*.

You have permission now to drop any lingering fear of salt, saturated fat, and cholesterol in your food. There's no need to gorge on butter, bacon, eggs, cheese, or fatty meats, but there's certainly no reason to avoid them either, especially if they come from grass-fed, foraging, or free-range animals. The "paradoxes" of populations with long, healthy lives in several countries where these foods have been consumed for centuries aren't paradoxes at all. Now that you've learned the truth about dietary fats, there's no mystery. The health of these populations has less to do with what they *are* eating—cheese, cream, and pâté in France, for example, or feta cheese and roasted lamb in Greece—and more to do with what they *aren't* eating: large amounts of highly processed industrial seed oils.

As this book comes to a close, let's take a moment to recap some key facts we've covered about omega-3 and omega-6 fats.

Omega-6 increases inflammation and oxidation

By consuming more omega-3 and less omega-6, you'll shift your body from a pro-inflammatory state to an anti-inflammatory state, cooling the fire of chronic inflammation that underlies so much of the chronic disease burden in the Western world.

Omega-6 increases cancer risk; omega-3 reduces risk

By competing for incorporation into your cell membranes, omega-3 fat helps to reduce the amount of omega-6 that becomes part of your cells. In particular, high doses of the long-chain omega-3s found in fatty fish may help reduce the uptake of linoleic acid into cancer cells and help reduce cancer growth. By consuming less omega-6 from industrial seed oils, you may be reducing your risk not only of developing cancer but also of promoting cancer growth.

Omega-3 reduces cardiovascular risk

Remember, omega-3 fats help reduce your risk of cardiovascular disease. These special fats have anti-inflammatory and pro-resolving effects in your body, lowering high blood pressure, reducing abnormal clotting, and facilitating proper function of your blood vessels.

Omega-6 increases your hunger and fat gain

Through limiting adulterated omega-6 fats in your diet, you can finally start curbing your hunger and start shedding extra pounds. Correcting your omega-6-to-omega-3 ratio will help your body more easily release excess stored fat.

Omega-3 increases muscle mass and speeds fat loss

The consumption of omega-3 fats can boost fat burning and help you build lean muscle—a win-win for achieving and maintaining a healthy weight. DHA in particular acts like a pacemaker in your cells: more DHA may raise your metabolic rate, increasing the number of calories you burn all the time, not just when you're exercising.

For your health as well as your children's health, and *their* children's health, get back to basics. Consume real, nutrient-dense foods as close as possible to the way nature created them. Use supplements strategically to correct any imbalances that you're not able to balance with food alone. You may not be able to control every aspect of your health, but you are in the driver's seat when it comes to using dietary fats to set the stage for good health now and in your future. All it requires is changing some of the foods you eat. We hope this book has shown you the way to do just that.

ENDNOTES

Introduction

1. Adapted from Enig, M. Know your fats. Silver Spring (MD): Bethesda Press; 2000. 358 p.

2. Fallon, S, Enig, M. The great con-ola [Internet]. Washington (DC): The Weston A. Price Foundation; 2002 Jul 28 [cited 2018 Jun 4]. Available from http://www.westonaprice.org/know-your-fats/the-great-con-ola/

3. Blasbalg TL, Hibbeln JR, Ramsden CE, et al. Changes in consumption of omega-3 and omega-6 fatty acids in the United States during the 20th century. *Am J Clin Nutr.* 2011 May;93(5):950-62.

4. Ibid.

5. Simopoulos AP. Essential fatty acids in health and chronic disease. *Am J Clin Nutr* 1999 Sep;70 (3 Suppl):560s-9s.

6. Simopoulos AP, DiNicolantonio JJ. The importance of a balanced omega-6 to omega-3 ratio in the prevention and management of obesity. *Open Heart.* 2016 Sep;3(2):e000385.

7. DiNicolantonio JJ, McCarty MF, Chatterjee S, et al. A higher dietary ratio of long-chain omega-3 to total omega-6 fatty acids for prevention of COX-2-dependent adenocarcinomas. *Nutr Cancer.* 2014;66(8):1279-84.

8. Simopoulos AP. Essential fatty acids in health and chronic disease. *Am J Clin Nutr.* 1999 Sep;70 (3 Suppl):560s-9s.

9. Kuipers RS, Luxwolda MF, Dijck-Brouwer DA, et al. Estimated macronutrient and fatty acid intakes from an East African Paleolithic diet. *Br J Nutr.* 2010 Dec;104(11):1666-87.

10. Singh RB, Demeester F, Wilczynska A. The tsim tsoum approaches for prevention of cardiovascular disease. *Cardiol Res Pract.* 2010;2010:824938.

11. Rodriguez-Leyva D, Dupasquier CM, McCullough R, et al. The cardiovascular effects of flaxseed and its omega-3 fatty acid, alpha-linolenic acid. *Can J Cardiol.* 2010 Nov;26(9):489-96.

12. Burdge GC, Wootton SA. Conversion of alpha-linolenic acid to eicosapentaenoic, docosapentaenoic and docosahexaenoic acids in young women. *Br J Nutr.* 2002 Oct;88(4):411-20.

13. Kuipers RS, Luxwolda MF, Dijck-Brouwer DA, et al. Estimated macronutrient and fatty acid intakes from an East African Paleolithic diet. *Br J Nutr.* 2010 Dec;104(11):1666-87.

14. Eaton SB, Eaton SB 3rd, Sinclair AJ, et al. Dietary intake of long-chain polyunsaturated fatty acids during the paleolithic. *World Rev Nutr Diet.* 1998;83:12-23.

Chapter 1

1. Keys A. Atherosclerosis: a problem in newer public health. *J Mt Sinai Hosp N Y.* 1953 Jul-Aug;20(2):118-39.

2. Yerushalmy J, Hilleboe HE. Fat in the diet and mortality from heart disease; a methodologic note. *N Y State J Med.* 1957 Jul 15;57(14):2343-54.

3. DiNicolantonio JJ, Lucan SC, O'Keefe JH. The evidence for saturated fat and for sugar related to coronary heart disease. *Prog Cardiovasc Dis.* 2016;58(5):464-72.

4. DiNicolantonio JJ. The cardiometabolic consequences of replacing saturated fats with carbohydrates or Ω-6 polyunsaturated fats: Do the dietary guidelines have it wrong? *Open Heart.* 2014 Feb 8;1(1):e000032. doi:10.1136/openhrt-2013 -000032.

5. Ahrens EH Jr., Insull W Jr., Blomstrand R, et al. The influence of dietary fats on serum-lipid levels in man. *Lancet.* 1957 May 11;272(6976):943-53.

6. Ahrens EH Jr., Blankenhorn DH, Tsaltas TT. Effect on human serum lipids of substituting plant for animal fat in diet. *Proc Soc Exp Biol Med.* 1954 Aug 1;86(4):872-8.

7. Parodi PW. Has the association between saturated fatty acids, serum cholesterol and coronary heart disease been over emphasized? *Intl Dairy J.* 2009 Jun-Jul;19(6-7):345-61.

8. Kannel WB, Dawber TR, Kagan A, et al. Factors of risk in the development of coronary heart disease--six year follow-up experience. The Framingham Study. *Ann Intern Med.* 1961 Jul;55:33-50.

9. Ramsden CE, Hibbeln JR, Majchrzak-Hong SF. All PUFAs are not created equal: absence of CHD benefit specific to linoleic acid in randomized controlled trials and prospective observational cohorts. *World Rev Nutr Diet.* 2011;102:30-43.

10. Mustad VA, Ellsworth JL, Cooper AD, et al. Dietary linoleic acid increases and palmitic acid decreases hepatic LDL receptor protein and mRNA abundance in young pigs. *J Lipid Res.* 1996 Nov;37(11):2310-23.

11. Ibid.

12. Fernandez ML, West KL. Mechanisms by which dietary fatty acids modulate plasma lipids. *J Nutr.* 2005 Sep;135(9):2075-8.

13. Dias CB, Garg R, Wood LG, et al. Saturated fat consumption may not be the main cause of increased blood lipid levels. *Med Hypotheses.* 2014 Feb;82(2):187-95.

14. Steinberg D. Thematic review series: the pathogenesis of atherosclerosis. An interpretive history of the cholesterol controversy, part V: the discovery of the statins and the end of the controversy. *J Lipid Res.* 2006 Jul;47(7):1339-51.

15. Parodi PW. Has the association between saturated fatty acids, serum cholesterol and coronary heart disease been over emphasized? *Intl Dairy J.* 2009 Jun-Jul;19(6-7):345-61.

16. Select Committee on Nutrition and Human Needs. Dietary goals for the United States [Internet]. Washington, DC: United States Senate; 1977 [cited 2018 Jul 15]. Available from http://zerodiseasecom/archive/Dietary_Goals_For_The_United_States.pdf.

17. Hu FB, Stampfer MJ, Manson JE, et al. Dietary fat intake and the risk of coronary heart disease in women. *N Engl J Med.* 1997;337(21):1491-9.

18. Oh K, Hu FB, Manson JE, et al. Dietary fat intake and risk of coronary heart disease in women: 20 years of follow-up of the nurses' health study. *Am J Epidemiol.* 2005 Apr 1;161(7):672-9.

19. Ramsden CE, Hibbeln JR, Majchrzak-Hong SF. All PUFAs are not created equal: absence of CHD benefit specific to linoleic acid in randomized controlled trials and prospective observational cohorts. *World Rev Nutr Diet.* 2011;102:30-43.

20. Huang X, Sjogren P, Arnlov J, et al. Serum fatty acid patterns, insulin sensitivity and the metabolic syndrome in individuals with chronic kidney disease. *J Intern Med.* 2014 Jan;275(1):71-83.

21. Wu JH, Lemaitre RN, King IB, et al. Circulating omega-6 polyunsaturated fatty acids and total and cause-specific mortality: the Cardiovascular Health Study. *Circulation.* 2014 Oct 7;130(15):1245-53.

22. Warensjo E, Sundstrom J, Vessby B, et al. Markers of dietary fat quality and fatty acid desaturation as predictors of total and cardiovascular mortality: a population-based prospective study. *Am J Clin Nutr.* 2008 Jul;88(1):203-9.

23. de Goede J, Verschuren WM, Boer JM, et al. N-6 and N-3 fatty acid cholesteryl esters in relation to fatal CHD in a Dutch adult population: a nested case-control study and meta-analysis. *PLoS One.* 2013 May 31;8(5):e59408.

24. Fernandez-Real JM, Broch M, Vendrell J, et al. Insulin resistance, inflammation, and serum fatty acid composition. *Diabetes Care.* 2003 May;26(5):1362-8.

25. Miettinen TA, Naukkarinen V, Huttunen JK, et al. Fatty-acid composition of serum lipids predicts myocardial infarction. *Br Med J (Clin Res Ed).* 1982 Oct 9;285(6347):993-6.

26. Wu JH, Lemaitre RN, King IB, et al. Circulating omega-6 polyunsaturated fatty acids and total and cause-specific mortality: the Cardiovascular Health Study. *Circulation.* 2014 Oct 7;130(15):1245-53.

27. Marventano S, Kolacz P, Castellano S, et al. A review of recent evidence in human studies of n-3 and n-6 PUFA intake on cardiovascular disease, cancer, and depressive disorders: does the ratio really matter? *Int J Food Sci Nutr.* 2015;66(6):611-22.

28. Keys A. Coronary heart disease in seven countries. 1970. *Nutrition.* 1997 Mar 13;13(3):250-2; discussion 49, 3.

29. Keys A. Mediterranean diet and public health: personal reflections. *Am J Clin Nutr.* 1995 Jun;61(6 Suppl):1321s-3s.

30. Ibid.

31. Dias CB, Garg R, Wood LG, et al. Saturated fat consumption may not be the main cause of increased blood lipid levels. *Med Hypotheses.* 2014 Feb;82(2):187-95.

32. Yano K, Rhoads GG, Kagan A, et al. Dietary intake and the risk of coronary heart disease in Japanese men living in Hawaii. *Am J Clin Nutr.* 1978 Jul;31(7):1270-9.

33. Ibid.

34. Keys A, Kimura N, Kusukawa A, et al. Lessons from serum cholesterol studies in Japan, Hawaii and Los Angeles. *Ann Intern Med.* 1958 Jan 1;48(1):83-94.

35. Parodi PW. Has the association between saturated fatty acids, serum cholesterol and coronary heart disease been over emphasized? *Int Dairy J.* 2009 Jun-Jul;19(6-7):345-61.

36. Ibid.

37. Ibid.

38. Ibid.

39. Ibid.

40. Campos H, Blijlevens E, McNamara JR, et al. LDL particle size distribution. Results from the Framingham Offspring Study. *Arterioscler Thromb.* 1992 Dec;12(1):1410-9.

41. Dreon DM, Fernstrom HA, Campos H, et al. Change in dietary saturated fat intake is correlated with change in mass of large low-density-lipoprotein particles in men. *Am J Clin Nutr.* 1998 May;67(5):828-36.

42. Parodi PW. Has the association between saturated fatty acids, serum cholesterol and coronary heart disease been over emphasized? *Int Dairy J.* 2009 (Jun-Jul;19(6-7):345-61.

43. Ibid.

44. Rizzo M, Berneis K. Low-density lipoprotein size and cardiovascular risk assessment. *QJM.* 2006 Jan;99(1):1-14.

45. Dreon DM, Fernstrom HA, Williams PT, et al. A very low-fat diet is not associated with improved lipoprotein profiles in men with a predominance of large, low-density lipoproteins. *Am J Clin Nutr.* 1999 Mar;69(3):411-8.

46. Turpeinen O, Karvonen MJ, Pekkarinen M, et al. Dietary prevention of coronary heart disease: the Finnish Mental Hospital Study. *Int J Epidemiol.* 1979 Jun;8(2):99-118.

47. Parodi PW. Has the association between saturated fatty acids, serum cholesterol and coronary heart disease been over emphasized? *Int Dairy J.* 2009 Jun-Jul;19(6-7):345-61.

48. Dayton S, Pearce ML. Diet high in unsaturated fat. A controlled clinical trial. *Minn Med.* 1969 Aug;52(8):1237-42.

49. Loffredo L, Perri L, Di Castelnuovo A, et al. Supplementation with vitamin E alone is associated with reduced myocardial infarction: a meta-analysis. *Nutr Metab Cardiovasc Dis.* 2015 Apr;25(4):354-63.

50. Ramsden CE, Hibbeln JR, Majchrzak SF, et al. n-6 fatty acid-specific and mixed polyunsaturate dietary interventions have different effects on CHD risk: a meta-analysis of randomised controlled trials. *Br J Nutr.* 2010 Dec;104(11):1586-600.

51. Ibid.

52. Frantz ID Jr., Dawson EA, Ashman PL, et al. Test of effect of lipid lowering by diet on cardiovascular risk. The Minnesota Coronary Survey. *Arteriosclerosis.* 1989 Jan-Feb;9(1):129-35.

53. Baum SJ, Kris-Etherton PM, Willett WC, et al. Fatty acids in cardiovascular health and disease: a comprehensive update. *J Clin Lipidol.* 2012 May-Jun;6(3):216-34.

54. Christakis G, Rinzler SH, Archer M, et al. Effect of the Anti-Coronary Club program on coronary heart disease. Risk-factor status. *JAMA.* 1966 Nov 7;198(6):597-604.

55. DiNicolantonio JJ. The cardiometabolic consequences of replacing saturated fats with carbohydrates or Ω-6 polyunsaturated fats: Do the dietary guidelines have it wrong? *Open Heart,* 2014 Feb 8;1(1):e000032. doi:10.1136/openhrt-2013 -000032.

56. Christakis G, Rinzler SH, Archer M, et al. The anti-coronary club. A dietary approach to the prevention of coronary heart disease—a seven-year report. *Am J Public Health Nations Health.* 1966 Feb;56(2):299-314.

57. Rose GA, Thomson WB, Williams RT. Corn oil in treatment of ischaemic heart disease. *Br Med J.* 1965 Jun 12;1(5449):1531-3.

58. Ibid.

59. De Lorgeril M, Salen P, Martin JL, et al. Mediterranean diet, traditional risk factors, and the rate of cardiovascular complications after myocardial infarction: final report of the Lyon Diet Heart Study. *Circulation.* 1999 Feb 16;99(6):779-85.

60. de Lorgeril M, Renaud S, Mamelle N, et al. Mediterranean alpha-linolenic acid-rich diet in secondary prevention of coronary heart disease. *Lancet.* 1994 Jun 11;343(8911):1454-9.

61. Estruch R, Ros E, Salas-Salvado J, et al. Primary prevention of cardiovascular disease with a Mediterranean diet. *N Engl J Med.* 2013 Apr 4;368(14):1279-90.

62. de Lorgeril M, Salen P, Defaye P, et al. Recent findings on the health effects of omega-3 fatty acids and statins, and their interactions: do statins inhibit omega-3? *BMC Med.* 2013;11:5.

63. DiNicolantonio JJ, Niazi AK, McCarty MF, et al. Omega-3s and cardiovascular health. *Ochsner J.* 2014 Fall;14(3):399-412.

64. DiNicolantonio JJ, Niazi AK, O'Keefe JH, Lavie CJ. Explaining the recent fish oil trial "failures". *J Glycomics Lipidomics.* 2013;3(1): e112. doi:10.4172/2153 -0637.1000e112.

65. Burr ML, Fehily AM, Gilbert JF, et al. Effects of changes in fat, fish, and fibre intakes on death and myocardial reinfarction: diet and reinfarction trial (DART). *Lancet.* 1989 Sep 30;2(8666):757-61.

66. Burr ML, Sweetham PM, Fehily AM. Diet and reinfarction. *Eur Heart J.* 1994 Aug;15(8):1152-3.

67. Marchioli R, Barzi F, Bomba E, et al. Early protection against sudden death by n-3 polyunsaturated fatty acids after myocardial infarction: time-course analysis of the results of the Gruppo Italiano per lo Studio della Sopravvivenza nell'Infarto Miocardico (GISSI)-Prevenzione. *Circulation.* 2002 Apr 23;105(16):1897-903.

68. Dietary supplementation with n-3 polyunsaturated fatty acids and vitamin E after myocardial infarction: results of the GISSI-Prevenzione trial. Gruppo Italiano per lo Studio della Sopravvivenza nell'Infarto miocardico. *Lancet.* 1999 Aug 7;354(9177):447-55.

69. Tavazzi L, Maggioni AP, Marchioli R, et al. Effect of n-3 polyunsaturated fatty acids in patients with chronic heart failure (the GISSI-HF trial): a randomised, double-blind, placebo-controlled trial. *Lancet.* 2008 Oct 4;372(9645):1223-30.

70. Yokoyama M, Origasa H, Matsuzaki M, et al. Effects of eicosapentaenoic acid on major coronary events in hypercholesterolaemic patients (JELIS): a randomised open-label, blinded endpoint analysis. *Lancet.* 2007 Mar 31;369(9567):1090-8.

71. Ibid.

72. Tanaka K, Ishikawa Y, Yokoyama M, et al. Reduction in the recurrence of stroke by eicosapentaenoic acid for hypercholesterolemic patients: subanalysis of the JELIS trial. *Stroke.* 2008 Jul;39(7):2052-8.

73. Einvik G, Klemsdal TO, Sandvik L, et al. A randomized clinical trial on n-3 polyunsaturated fatty acids supplementation and all-cause mortality in elderly men at high cardiovascular risk. *Eur J Cardiovasc Prev Rehabil.* 2010 Oct;17(5):588-92.

74. Simopoulos AP. The importance of the ratio of omega-6/omega-3 essential fatty acids. *Biomed Pharmacother.* 2002 Oct;56(8):365-79.

75. DiNicolantonio JJ, Meier P, O'Keefe JH. Omega-3 polyunsaturated fatty acids for the prevention of cardiovascular disease: do formulation, dosage & comparator matter? *Mo Med.* 2013 Nov-Dec;110(6):495-8.

76. Simopoulos AP, Leaf A, Salem N Jr. Essentiality of and recommended dietary intakes for omega-6 and omega-3 fatty acids. *Ann Nutr Metab.* 1999;43(2):127-30.

77. Harris WS, Von Schacky C. The omega-3 index: a new risk factor for death from coronary heart disease? *Prev Med.* 2004 Jul;39(1):212-20.

Chapter 2

1. Lee KW, Lee HJ, Cho HY, et al. Role of the conjugated linoleic acid in the prevention of cancer. *Crit Rev Food Sci Nutr.* 2005;45(2):135-44.

2. Wang Y, Lu J, Ruth MR, et al. Trans-11 vaccenic acid dietary supplementation induces hypolipidemic effects in JCR:LA-cp rats. *J Nutr.* 2008 Nov;138(1):2117-22.

3. Micha R, Mozaffarian D. Trans fatty acids: effects on cardiometabolic health and implications for policy. *Prostaglandins Leukot Essent Fatty Acids*. 2008;79(3-5):147-52.

4. Kinsella JE, Bruckner G, Mai J, et al. Metabolism of trans fatty acids with emphasis on the effects of trans, trans-octadecadienoate on lipid composition, essential fatty acid, and prostaglandins: an overview. *Am J Clin Nutr*. 1981 Oct;34(1):2307-18.

5. Tardy AL, Morio B, Chardigny JM, et al. Ruminant and industrial sources of trans-fat and cardiovascular and diabetic diseases. *Nut Res Rev*. 2011 Jun;24(1):111-7.

6. Morris MC, Evans DA, Bienias JL, et al. Dietary fats and the risk of incident Alzheimer disease. *Arch Neurol*. 2003 Feb;60(2):194-200.

7. Chavarro JE, Stampfer MJ, Campos H, et al. A prospective study of trans-fatty acid levels in blood and risk of prostate cancer. *Cancer Epidemiol Biomarkers Prev*. 2008 Jan;17(1):95-101.

8. Chajes V, Thiebaut AC, Rotival M, et al. Association between serum trans-monounsaturated fatty acids and breast cancer risk in the E3N-EPIC Study. *Am J Epidemiol*. 2008 Jun 1;167(11):1312-20.

9. Phivilay A, Julien C, Tremblay C, et al. High dietary consumption of trans fatty acids decreases brain docosahexaenoic acid but does not alter amyloid-beta and tau pathologies in the 3xTg-AD model of Alzheimer's disease. *Neuroscience*. 2009 Mar 3;159(1):296-307.

10. Golomb BA, Bui AK. A fat to forget: trans fat consumption and memory. *PLoS One*. 2015 Jun 17;10(6):e0128129.

11. Sanchez-Villegas A, Verberne L, De Irala J, et al. Dietary fat intake and the risk of depression: the SUN Project. *PLoS One*. 2011 Jan 26;6(1):e16268.

12. A scientific discovery which will affect every kitchen in America. *Ladies Home Journal*. 2012:45. Available from https://hdl.handle.net/2027/mdp .39015011414177?urlappend=%3Bseq=53.1177-9.

13. Rupp, R. The butter wars: when margarine was pink [Internet]. *Nat Geographic*. 2014 Aug 13 [cited 4 June 2018]. Available from http://theplate. nationalgeographic.com/2014/08/13/the-butter-wars-when-margarine-was -pink/.

14. Braun, AD. Turning bacon into bombs [Internet]. *Atlantic*. 2014 Apr 18 [cited 4 June 2018]. Available from http://www.theatlantic.com/health/archive/2014/04 /reluctantly-turning-bacon-into-bombs-during-world-war-ii/360298/.

15. History of the American Heart Association [Internet]. *Am Heart Assn*. [cited 4 June 2018]. Available from http://www.heart.org/HEARTORG/General /History-of-the-American-Heart-Association_UCM_308120_Article .jsp?appName=MobileApp.

16. Enig, M, Fallon S. Eat fat, lose fat: the healthy alternative to trans fats. New York (NY): Penguin; 2004. 304 p.

17. Christakis, G. The anti-coronary club. A dietary approach to the prevention of coronary heath disease: a seven-year report. *Am J Pub Health*. 1966 Feb;56(2):299-314. Available from http://www.epi.umn.edu/cvdepi/study -synopsis/anti-coronary-club-trial/.

18. Christakis G, Rinzler SH, Archer M, et al. Effect of the Anti-Coronary Club program on coronary heart disease. Risk-factor status. *JAMA*. 1966 Nov 7;198(6):597-604.

19. Johnston PV, Johnson OC, Kummerow FA. Occurrence of trans fatty acids in human tissue. *Science*. 1957 Oct 11;126(3296):698-9.

20. Kummerow FA, et al. The influence of three sources of dietary fats and cholesterol on lipid composition of swine serum lipids and aorta tissue. *Artery 4*. 1978:360-384.

21. Schleifer D. We spent a million bucks and then we had to do something: the unexpected implications of industry involvement in trans fat research [Internet]. *Bull of Science, Tech & Soc*. 2011 Oct 4 [cited 4 June 2018];31(6):460-471. Available from http://journals.sagepub.com/doi /abs/10.1177/0270467611422837

22. Guidance for industry: trans fatty acids in nutrition labeling, nutrient content claims, health claims; small entity compliance guide [Internet]. *FDA*. 2018 Aug [cited 4 June 2018]. Available from http://www.fda.gov/RegulatoryInformation /Guidances/ucm053479.htm.

23. AMA supports ban of artificial trans fats in restaurants and bakeries nationwide. *AMA*. 2008 Press release, 2008 Nov 10 [accessed 2 June 2009]. Available from http://www.ama-assn.org/ama/pub/category/20273.html.

24. United States military casualties of war [Internet]. *Wikipedia*. 2018 May 21 [cited 4 June 2018]. Available from https://en.wikipedia.org/wiki/United_States _military_casualties_of_war.

Chapter 3

1. Leaf A, Weber PC. A new era for science in nutrition. *Am J Clin Nutr*. 1987 May;45(5 Suppl):1048-53.

2. Ibid.

3. Singh RB, Demeester F, Wilczynska A. The tsim tsoum approaches for prevention of cardiovascular disease. *Cardiol Res Pract*. 2010;2010:824938.

4. Ibid.

5. Kuipers RS, Luxwolda MF, Dijck-Brouwer DA, et al. Estimated macronutrient and fatty acid intakes from an East African Paleolithic diet. *Br J Nutr*. 2010 Dec;104(11):1666-87.

6. Sprecher H. Dietary w3 and w6 fatty acids: biological effects and nutritional essentiality. *NATO Series A, Life Sciences*. 1989 Jan:69-79.

7. Peskin B. Plants vs. fish: why plants win. *Aging Matters Magazine*. 2015;1:6-11.

8. Kemsley T. Animal brains a favorite among early humans: a study [Internet]. *Nature World News*. 2013 May 6 [cited 4 June 2018]. Available from http:// www.natureworldnews.com/articles/1765/20130506/animal-brains-favorite -early-humans-study.htm.

9. Cordain L, Watkins BA, Florant GL, et al. Fatty acid analysis of wild ruminant tissues: evolutionary implications for reducing diet-related chronic disease. *Eur J Clin Nutr*. 2002 Mar;56(3):181-91.

10. Ferraro JV, Plummer TW, Pobiner BL, et al. Earliest archaeological evidence of persistent hominin carnivory. *PLoS One.* 2013 Apr 25;8(4):e62174.

11. Eaton SB, Eaton SB 3rd, Sinclair AJ, et al. Dietary intake of long-chain polyunsaturated fatty acids during the paleolithic. *World Rev Nutr Diet.* 1998;83:12-23.

12. Kuipers RS, Luxwolda MF, Dijck-Brouwer DA, et al. Estimated macronutrient and fatty acid intakes from an East African Paleolithic diet. *Br J Nutr.* 2010 Dec;104(11):1666-87.

13. Mathias RA, Fu W, Akey JM, et al. Adaptive evolution of the FADS gene cluster within Africa. *PLoS One.* 2012;7(9):e44926.

14. Kuipers RS, Luxwolda MF, Dijck-Brouwer DA, et al. Estimated macronutrient and fatty acid intakes from an East African Paleolithic diet. *Br J Nutr.* 2010 Dec;104(11):1666-87.

15. Plourde M, Cunnane SC. Extremely limited synthesis of long chain polyunsaturates in adults: implications for their dietary essentiality and use as supplements. *Appl Phys Nutr Metab.* 2007 Aug;32(4):619-34.

16. Leaf A, Weber PC. A new era for science in nutrition. *Am J Clin Nutr.* 1987 May;45(5 Suppl):1048-53.

17. Eaton SB, Konner M. Paleolithic nutrition. A consideration of its nature and current implications. *N Engl J Med.* 1985 Jan 31;312(5):283-9.

18. Cordain L, Watkins BA, Florant GL, et al. Fatty acid analysis of wild ruminant tissues: evolutionary implications for reducing diet-related chronic disease. *Eur J Clin Nutr.* 2002 Mar;56(3):181-91.

19. Sprecher H. Dietary w3 and w6 fatty acids: biological effects and nutritional essentiality. *NATO Series A, Life Sciences.* 1989 Jan:69-79.

20. Ibid.

21. Cordain L, Watkins BA, Florant GL, et al. Fatty acid analysis of wild ruminant tissues: evolutionary implications for reducing diet-related chronic disease. *Eur J Clin Nutr.* 2002 Mar;56(3):181-91.

22. Ibid.

23. Singh RB, Demeester F, Wilczynska A. The tsim tsoum approaches for prevention of cardiovascular disease. *Cardiol Res Pract.* 2010;2010:824938.

24. Ibid.

25. Eaton SB, Eaton SB 3rd, Sinclair AJ, et al. Dietary intake of long-chain polyunsaturated fatty acids during the paleolithic. *World Rev Nutr Diet.* 1998;83:12-23.

26. Kris-Etherton PM, Taylor DS, Yu-Poth S, et al. Polyunsaturated fatty acids in the food chain in the United States. *Am J Clin Nutr.* 2000 Jan;71(1 Suppl):179s-88s.

27. Singh RB, Demeester F, Wilczynska A. The tsim tsoum approaches for prevention of cardiovascular disease. *Cardiol Res Pract.* 2010;2010:824938.

28. Rodriguez-Leyva D, Dupasquier CM, McCullough R, et al. The cardiovascular effects of flaxseed and its omega-3 fatty acid, alpha-linolenic acid. *Can J Cardiol.* 2010 Nov;26(9):489-96.

29. Kuipers RS, Luxwolda MF, Dijck-Brouwer DA, et al. Estimated macronutrient and fatty acid intakes from an East African Paleolithic diet. *Br J Nutr.* 2010 Dec;104(11):1666-87.

30. Eaton SB, Eaton SB 3rd, Sinclair AJ, et al. Dietary intake of long-chain polyunsaturated fatty acids during the paleolithic. *World Rev Nutr Diet.* 1998;83:12-23.

31. Peskin B. Plants vs. fish: why plants win. *Aging Matters Magazine.* 2015;1:6-11.

32. Ramsden CE, Ringel A, Feldstein AE, et al. Lowering dietary linoleic acid reduces bioactive oxidized linoleic acid metabolites in humans. *Prostaglandins Leukot Essent Fatty Acids.* 2012 Oct-Nov;87(4-5):135-41.

33. Singh RB, Demeester F, Wilczynska A. The tsim tsoum approaches for prevention of cardiovascular disease. *Cardiol Res Pract.* 2010;2010:824938.

34. Kuipers RS, Luxwolda MF, Dijck-Brouwer DA, et al. Estimated macronutrient and fatty acid intakes from an East African Paleolithic diet. *Br J Nutr.* 2010 Dec;104 (11):1666-87.

35. Eaton SB, Eaton SB 3rd, Sinclair AJ, et al. Dietary intake of long-chain polyunsaturated fatty acids during the paleolithic. *World Rev Nutr Diet.* 1998;83:12-23.

36. Kris-Etherton PM, Taylor DS, Yu-Poth S, et al. Polyunsaturated fatty acids in the food chain in the United States. *Am J Clin Nutr.* 2000 Jan;71(1 Suppl):179s-88s.

37. Singh RB, Demeester F, Wilczynska A. The tsim tsoum approaches for prevention of cardiovascular disease. *Cardiol Res Pract.* 2010;2010:824938.

38. Kuipers RS, Luxwolda MF, Dijck-Brouwer DA, et al. Estimated macronutrient and fatty acid intakes from an East African Paleolithic diet. *Br J Nutr.* 2010 Dec;104(11):1666-87.

39. Rodriguez-Leyva D, Dupasquier CM, McCullough R, et al. The cardiovascular effects of flaxseed and its omega-3 fatty acid, alpha-linolenic acid. *Can J Cardiol.* 2010 Nov;26(9):489-96.

40. Kuipers RS, Luxwolda MF, Dijck-Brouwer DA, et al. Estimated macronutrient and fatty acid intakes from an East African Paleolithic diet. *Br J Nutr.* 2010 Dec;104(11):1666-87.

41. Eaton SB, Eaton SB 3rd, Sinclair AJ, et al. Dietary intake of long-chain polyunsaturated fatty acids during the paleolithic. *World Rev Nutr Diet.* 1998;83:12-23.

42. Singh RB, Demeester F, Wilczynska A. The tsim tsoum approaches for prevention of cardiovascular disease. *Cardiol Res Pract.* 2010;2010:824938.

43. Rodriguez-Leyva D, Dupasquier CM, McCullough R, et al. The cardiovascular effects of flaxseed and its omega-3 fatty acid, alpha-linolenic acid. *Can J Cardiol.* 2010 Nov;26(9):489-96.

44. Kuipers RS, Luxwolda MF, Dijck-Brouwer DA, et al. Estimated macronutrient and fatty acid intakes from an East African Paleolithic diet. *Br J Nutr.* 2010 Dec;104(11):1666-87.

45. Ibid.

46. DeFilippis AP, Sperling LS. Understanding omega-3's. *Am Heart J.* 2006 Mar;151(3):564-70.

47. Kuipers RS, Luxwolda MF, Dijck-Brouwer DA, et al. Estimated macronutrient and fatty acid intakes from an East African Paleolithic diet. *Br J Nutr.* 2010 Dec;104(11):1666-87.

48. Hite AH, Feinman RD, Guzman GE, et al. In the face of contradictory evidence: report of the Dietary Guidelines for Americans Committee. *Nutrition.* 2010 Oct;26(1):915-24.

49. Wells, HF, Buzby JC. Dietary assessment of major trends in U.S. food consumption, 1970-2005. *ERS Report Summary.* 2008 Mar.

50. Food labeling: trans fatty acids in nutrition labeling, nutrient content claims, and health claims. Final rule. *Fed Regist.* 2003 Jul 11;68(133):41433-1506.

Chapter 4

1. Simopoulos AP. The importance of the omega-6/omega-3 fatty acid ratio in cardiovascular disease and other chronic diseases. *Exp Biol Med (Maywood).* 2008 Jun;233(6):674-88.

2. Simopoulos AP. The importance of the ratio of omega-6/omega-3 essential fatty acids. *Biomed Pharmacother.* 2002 Oct;56(8):365-79.

3. Ibid.

4. Leaf A, Weber PC. A new era for science in nutrition. *Am J Clin Nutr.* 1987 May;45(5 Suppl):1048-53.

5. Ibid.

6. Simopoulos AP. The importance of the ratio of omega-6/omega-3 essential fatty acids. *Biomed Pharmacother.* 2002 Oct;56(8):365-79.

7. Leaf A, Weber PC. A new era for science in nutrition. *Am J Clin Nutr.* 1987 May;45(5 Suppl):1048-53.

8. Sperling LS, Nelson JR. History and future of omega-3 fatty acids in cardiovascular disease. *Curr Med Res Opin.* 2016;32(2):301-11.

9. Kromann N, Green A. Epidemiological studies in the Upernavik district, Greenland. Incidence of some chronic diseases 1950-1974. *Acta Med Scand.* 1980 Jan-Dec;208:401-6.

10. Okuyama H, Kobayashi T, Watanabe S. Dietary fatty acids—the N-6/N-3 balance and chronic elderly diseases. Excess linoleic acid and relative N-3 deficiency syndrome seen in Japan. *Prog Lipid Res.* 1996 Dec;35(4):409-57.

11. Ibid.

12. Ibid.

13. Ibid.

14. Imaida K, Sato H, Okamiya H, et al. Enhancing effect of high fat diet on 4-nitroquinoline 1-oxide-induced pulmonary tumorigenesis in ICR male mice. *Jpn J Cancer Res.* 1989 Jun;80(6):499-502.

15. Okuyama H, Kobayashi T, Watanabe S. Dietary fatty acids—the N-6/N-3 balance and chronic elderly diseases. Excess linoleic acid and relative N-3 deficiency syndrome seen in Japan. *Prog Lipid Res.* 1996 Dec;35(4):409-57.

16. Ibid.

17. Ibid.

18. Ibid.

19. Malhotra SL. Epidemiology of ischaemic heart disease in India with special reference to causation. *Br Heart J.* 1967 Nov;29(6):895-905.

20. Ibid.

21. Padmavati S. Epidemiology of cardiovascular disease in India. II. Ischemic heart disease. *Circulation.* 1962 Apr;25:711-7.

22. Malhotra SL. Epidemiology of ischaemic heart disease in India with special reference to causation. *Br Heart J.* 1967 Nov;29(6):895-905.

23. Ibid.

24. Ibid.

25. Ibid.

26. Ibid.

27. Ghee [Internet]. *Wikipedia.* 2018 May 21 [cited 4 Jun 2018]. Available from https://en.wikipedia.org/wiki/Ghee.

28. Padmavati S. Epidemiology of cardiovascular disease in India. II. Ischemic heart disease. *Circulation.* 1962 Apr;25:711-7.

29. Malhotra SL. Geographical aspects of acute myocardial infarction in India with special reference to patterns of diet and eating. *Br Heart J.* 1967 May;29(3):337-44.

30. Padmavati S. Epidemiology of cardiovascular disease in India. II. Ischemic heart disease. *Circulation.* 1962 Apr;25:711-7.

31. Ibid.

32. Ibid.

33. Raheja BS, Sadikot SM, Phatak RB, et al. Significance of the N-6/N-3 ratio for insulin action in diabetes. *Ann N Y Acad Sci.* 1993 Jun 14;683:258-71.

34. Ibid.

35. Ibid.

36. Lindeberg S, Nilsson-Ehle P, Vessby B. Lipoprotein composition and serum cholesterol ester fatty acids in nonwesternized Melanesians. *Lipids.* 1996 Feb;31(2):153-8.

37. Ibid.

38. Esposito K, Marfella R, Ciotola M, et al. Effect of a mediterranean-style diet on endothelial dysfunction and markers of vascular inflammation in the metabolic syndrome: a randomized trial. *JAMA.* 2004 Sep 22;292(12):1440-6.

39. Ibid.

40. Singh RB, Demeester F, Wilczynska A. The tsim tsoum approaches for prevention of cardiovascular disease. *Cardiol Res Pract.* 2010;2010:824938.

41. Adapted from Singh RB, Demeester F, Wilczynska A. The tsim tsoum approaches for prevention of cardiovascular disease. *Cardiol Res Pract.* 2010;2010:824938.

42. Massaro M, Habib A, Lubrano L, et al. The omega-3 fatty acid docosahexaenoate attenuates endothelial cyclooxygenase-2 induction through both NADP(H) oxidase and PKC epsilon inhibition. *Proc Natl Acad Sci U S A.* 2006 Oct 10;103(41):15184-9.

43. Sun Q, Ma J, Campos H, et al. Comparison between plasma and erythrocyte fatty acid content as biomarkers of fatty acid intake in US women. *Am J Clin Nutr.* 2007 Jul;86(1):74-81.

44. Grenon SM, Conte MS, Nosova E, et al. Association between n-3 polyunsaturated fatty acid content of red blood cells and inflammatory biomarkers in patients with peripheral artery disease. *J Vasc Surg.* 2013 Nov;58(5):1283-90.

45. Harris WS. The omega-3 index as a risk factor for coronary heart disease. *Am J Clin Nutr.* 2008 Jun;87(6):1997s-2002s.

46. Farzaneh-Far R, Harris WS, Garg S, et al. Inverse association of erythrocyte n-3 fatty acid levels with inflammatory biomarkers in patients with stable coronary artery disease: The Heart and Soul Study. *Atherosclerosis.* 2009 Aug;205(2):538-43.

Chapter 5

1. Pope AJ, Druhan L, Guzman JE, et al. Role of DDAH-1 in lipid peroxidation product-mediated inhibition of endothelial NO generation. *Am J Physiol Cell Physiol.* 2007 Nov;293(5):C1679-86.

2. Ibid.

3. Chen L, Zhou JP, Kuang DB, et al. 4-HNE increases intracellular ADMA levels in cultured HUVECs: evidence for miR-21-dependent mechanisms. *PLoS One.* 2013 May 22;8(5):e64148.

4. Yla-Herttuala S, Palinski W, Rosenfeld ME, et al. Evidence for the presence of oxidatively modified low density lipoprotein in atherosclerotic lesions of rabbit and man. *J Clin Invest.* 1989 Oct;84(4):1086-95.

5. Lahoz C, Alonso R, Ordovas JM, et al. Effects of dietary fat saturation on eicosanoid production, platelet aggregation and blood pressure. *Eur J Clin Invest.* 1997 Sep;27(9):780-7.

6. Gradinaru D, Borsa C, Ionescu C, et al. Oxidized LDL and NO synthesis—Biomarkers of endothelial dysfunction and ageing. *Mech Ageing Dev.* 2015 Nov;151:101-13.

7. Bonaa KH, Bjerve KS, Straume B, et al. Effect of eicosapentaenoic and docosahexaenoic acids on blood pressure in hypertension. A population-based intervention trial from the Tromso study. *N Engl J Med.* 1990;322:795-801.

8. Ibid.

9. Ferrara LA, Raimondi AS, d'Episcopo L, et al. Olive oil and reduced need for antihypertensive medications. *Arch Intern Med.* 2000 Mar 27;160(6):837-42.

10. Ibid.

11. Ibid.

12. Pope AJ, Druhan L, Guzman JE, et al. Role of DDAH-1 in lipid peroxidation product-mediated inhibition of endothelial NO generation. *Am J Physiol Cell Physiol.* 2007 Nov;293(5):C1679-86.

13. Wang XL, Zhang L, Youker K, et al. Free fatty acids inhibit insulin signaling-stimulated endothelial nitric oxide synthase activation through upregulating PTEN or inhibiting Akt kinase. *Diabetes.* 2006 Aug;55(8):2301-10.

14. Gradinaru D, Borsa C, Ionescu C, et al. Oxidized LDL and NO synthesis—Biomarkers of endothelial dysfunction and ageing. *Mech Ageing Dev.* 2015 Nov;151:101-13.

15. Lahoz C, Alonso R, Ordovas JM, et al. Effects of dietary fat saturation on eicosanoid production, platelet aggregation and blood pressure. *Eur J Clin Invest.* 1997 Sep;27(9):780-7.

16. Marchix J, Choque B, Kouba M, et al. Excessive dietary linoleic acid induces proinflammatory markers in rats. *J Nutr Biochem.* 2015 Dec;26(12):1434-41.

17. Hennig B, Toborek M, McClain CJ. High-energy diets, fatty acids and endothelial cell function: implications for atherosclerosis. *J Am Coll Nutr.* 2001 Apr;20(2 Suppl):97-105.

18. Simpson HC, Mann JI, Meade TW, et al. Hypertriglyceridaemia and hypercoagulability. *Lancet* 1983 Apr 9;1(8328):786-90.

19. Yosefy C, Viskoper JR, Laszt A, et al. The effect of fish oil on hypertension, plasma lipids and hemostasis in hypertensive, obese, dyslipidemic patients with and without diabetes mellitus. *Prostaglandins Leukot Essent Fatty Acids.* 1999 Aug;61(2):83-7.

20. Morris MC, Sacks F, Rosner B. Does fish oil lower blood pressure? A meta-analysis of controlled trials. *Circulation.* 1993 Aug 1;88(2):523-33.

21. Appel LJ, Miller ER 3rd, Seidler AJ, et al. Does supplementation of diet with 'fish oil' reduce blood pressure? A meta-analysis of controlled clinical trials. *Arch Intern Med.* 1993 Jun 28;153(12):1429-38.

22. Geleijnse JM, Giltay EJ, Grobbee DE, et al. Blood pressure response to fish oil supplementation: metaregression analysis of randomized trials. *J Hypertens.* 2002 Aug;20(8):1493-9.

23. Wang Q, Liang X, Wang L, et al. Effect of omega-3 fatty acids supplementation on endothelial function: a meta-analysis of randomized controlled trials. *Atherosclerosis.* 2012 Apr;221(2):536-43.

24. Egert S, Stehle P. Impact of n-3 fatty acids on endothelial function: results from human interventions studies. *Curr Opin Clin Nutr Metab Care.* 2011 Mar;14(2):121-31.

25. Berry EM, Hirsch J. Does dietary linolenic acid influence blood pressure? *Am J Clin Nutr.* 1986 Sep;44(3):336-40.

26. Griffin MD, Sanders TA, Davies IG, et al. Effects of altering the ratio of dietary n-6 to n-3 fatty acids on insulin sensitivity, lipoprotein size, and postprandial lipemia in men and postmenopausal women aged 45-70 y: the OPTILIP Study. *Am J Clin Nutr.* 2006 Dec;84(6):1290-8.

27. Hartwich J, Malec MM, Partyka L, et al. The effect of the plasma n-3/n-6 polyunsaturated fatty acid ratio on the dietary LDL phenotype transformation — Insights from the LIPGENE study. *Clin Nutr.* 2009 Oct;28(5):510-5.

28. Ibid.

29. Calabresi L, Donati D, Pazzucconi F, et al. Omacor in familial combined hyperlipidemia: effects on lipids and low density lipoprotein subclasses. *Atherosclerosis.* 2000 Feb;148(2):387-96.

30. Ibid.

31. Egert S, Kannenberg F, Somoza V, et al. Dietary alpha-linolenic acid, EPA, and DHA have differential effects on LDL fatty acid composition but similar effects on serum lipid profiles in normolipidemic humans. *J Nutr.* 2009 May;139(5):861-8.

32. Wilkinson P, Leach C, Ah-Sing EE, et al. Influence of alpha-linolenic acid and fish-oil on markers of cardiovascular risk in subjects with an atherogenic lipoprotein phenotype. *Atherosclerosis.* 2005 Jul;181(1):115-24.

33. Ibid.

34. Mori TA, Burke V, Puddey IB, et al. Purified eicosapentaenoic and docosahexaenoic acids have differential effects on serum lipids and lipoproteins, LDL particle size, glucose, and insulin in mildly hyperlipidemic men. *Am J Clin Nutr.* 2000 May;71(5):1085-94.

35. Kelley DS, Siegel D, Vemuri M, et al. Docosahexaenoic acid supplementation improves fasting and postprandial lipid profiles in hypertriglyceridemic men. *Am J Clin Nutr.* 2007 Aug;86(2):324-33.

36. Egert S, Kannenberg F, Somoza V, et al. Dietary alpha-linolenic acid, EPA, and DHA have differential effects on LDL fatty acid composition but similar effects on serum lipid profiles in normolipidemic humans. *J Nutr.* 2009 May;139(5):861-8.

37. Buckley R, Shewring B, Turner R, et al. Circulating triacylglycerol and apoE levels in response to EPA and docosahexaenoic acid supplementation in adult human subjects. *Br J Nutr.* 2004 Sep;92(3):477-83.

38. Nestel P, Shige H, Pomeroy S, et al. The n-3 fatty acids eicosapentaenoic acid and docosahexaenoic acid increase systemic arterial compliance in humans. *Am J Clin Nutr.* 2002 Aug;76(2):326-30.

39. Mori TA, Woodman RJ. The independent effects of eicosapentaenoic acid and docosahexaenoic acid on cardiovascular risk factors in humans. *Curr Opin Clin Nutr Metab Care.* 2006 Mar;9(2):95-104.

40. Din JN, Harding SA, Valerio CJ, et al. Dietary intervention with oil rich fish reduces platelet-monocyte aggregation in man. *Atherosclerosis.* 2008 Mar;197(1):290-6.

41. Harris WS. Expert opinion: omega-3 fatty acids and bleeding—cause for concern? *Am J Cardiol.* 2007 Mar 19;99(6A):44c-6c.

42. Olsen SF, Sorensen JD, Secher NJ, et al. Randomised controlled trial of effect of fish-oil supplementation on pregnancy duration. *Lancet.* 1992 Apr 25;339(8800):1003-7.

43. Harris WS. Expert opinion: omega-3 fatty acids and bleeding—cause for concern? *Am J Cardiol.* 2007 Mar 19;99(6A):44c-6c.

44. Reiffel JA, McDonald A. Antiarrhythmic effects of omega-3 fatty acids. *Am J Cardiol.* 2006 Aug 21;98(4A):50i-60i.

45. AHA releases 2015 heart and stroke statistics [Internet]. *SCA News.* 2014 Dec 30 [cited 4 Jun 2018]. Available from http://www.sca-aware.org/sca-news/aha -releases-2015-heart-and-stroke-statistics.

46. Sudden cardiac arrest [Internet]. *SCA News* [cited 4 Jun 2018]. Available from http://www.sca-aware.org/about-sca.

47. Marchioli R, Barzi F, Bomba E, et al. Early protection against sudden death by n-3 polyunsaturated fatty acids after myocardial infarction: time-course analysis of the results of the Gruppo Italiano per lo Studio della Sopravvivenza nell'Infarto Miocardico (GISSI)-Prevenzione. *Circulation.* 2002 Apr 23;105(16):1897-903.

48. De Backer G, Ambrosioni E, Borch-Johnsen K, et al. European guidelines on cardiovascular disease prevention in clinical practice. Third Joint Task Force of European and Other Societies on cardiovascular disease prevention in clinical practice. *Eur Heart J.* 2003 Sep;24(17):1601-10.

49. Marchioli R, Barzi F, Bomba E, et al. Early protection against sudden death by n-3 polyunsaturated fatty acids after myocardial infarction: time-course analysis of the results of the Gruppo Italiano per lo Studio della Sopravvivenza nell'Infarto Miocardico (GISSI)-Prevenzione. *Circulation.* 2002 Apr 23;105(16):1897-903.

50. Reiffel JA, McDonald A. Antiarrhythmic effects of omega-3 fatty acids. *Am J Cardiol.* 2006 Aug 21;98(4A):50i-60i.

51. von Schacky C. Cardiovascular disease prevention and treatment. *Prostaglandins Leukot Essent Fatty Acids.* 2009 Aug-Sep;81(2-3):193-8.

52. Ibid.

53. Itomura M, Fujioka S, Hamazaki K, et al. Factors influencing EPA+DHA levels in red blood cells in Japan. *In Vivo.* 2008 Jan-Feb;22(1):131-5.

54. Harris WS, Von Schacky C. The omega-3 index: a new risk factor for death from coronary heart disease? *Prev Med.* 2004 Jul;39:212-20.

55. von Schacky C, Harris WS. Cardiovascular benefits of omega-3 fatty acids. *Cardiovasc Res.* 2007 Jan 15;73(2):310-5.

56. Siscovick DS, Raghunathan TE, King I, et al. Dietary intake and cell membrane levels of long-chain n-3 polyunsaturated fatty acids and the risk of primary cardiac arrest. *JAMA.* 1995 Nov 1;274(17):1363-7.

57. Zampelas A, Roche H, Knapper JM, et al. Differences in postprandial lipaemic response between Northern and Southern Europeans. *Atherosclerosis.* 1998 Jul;139(1):83-93.

58. Perez-Jimenez F, Lopez-Miranda J, Mata P. Protective effect of dietary monounsaturated fat on arteriosclerosis: beyond cholesterol. *Atherosclerosis.* 2002 Aug;163(2):385-98.

59. Dubnov G, Berry EM. Omega-6/omega-3 fatty acid ratio: the Israeli paradox. *World Rev Nutr Diet.* 2003;92:81-91.

60. Yam D, Eliraz A, Berry EM. Diet and disease—the Israeli paradox: possible dangers of a high omega-6 polyunsaturated fatty acid diet. *Isr J Med Sci.* 1996 Nov;32(11):1134-43.

61. Renaud S, de Lorgeril M, Delaye J, et al. Cretan Mediterranean diet for prevention of coronary heart disease. *Am J Clin Nutr.* 1995 Jun 1;61(6):1360s-7s.

62. Covas MI, Nyyssonen K, Poulsen HE, et al. The effect of polyphenols in olive oil on heart disease risk factors: a randomized trial. *Ann Intern Med.* 2006 Sep 5;145(5):333-41.

63. Ibid.

64. Is your olive oil fake? [Internet]. *Mercola.com.* 2016 Dec 17 [cited 4 Jun 2018]. Available from https://articles.mercola.com/sites/articles/archive/2016/12/17/fake-olive-oil.aspx.

Chapter 6

1. Borkman M, Storlien LH, Pan DA, et al. The relation between insulin sensitivity and the fatty-acid composition of skeletal-muscle phospholipids. *N Engl J Med.* 1993 Jan 28;328(4):238-44.

2. Vessby B, Gustafsson IB, Tengblad S, et al. Desaturation and elongation of fatty acids and insulin action. *Ann N Y Acad Sci.* 2002 Jun;967:183-95.

3. de Lorgeril M, Salen P, Defaye P, et al. Recent findings on the health effects of omega-3 fatty acids and statins, and their interactions: do statins inhibit omega-3? *BMC Med.* 2013;11:5.

4. Rise P, Ghezzi S, Priori I, et al. Differential modulation by simvastatin of the metabolic pathways in the n-9, n-6 and n-3 fatty acid series, in human monocytic and hepatocytic cell lines. *Biochem Pharmacol.* 2005 Apr 1;69(7):1095-100.

5. de Lorgeril M, Salen P, Guiraud A, et al. Lipid-lowering drugs and essential omega-6 and omega-3 fatty acids in patients with coronary heart disease. *Nutr Metab Cardiovasc Dis.* 2005 Feb;15(1):36-41.

6. Nozue T, Yamamoto S, Tohyama S, et al. Comparison of effects of serum n-3 to n-6 polyunsaturated fatty acid ratios on coronary atherosclerosis in patients treated with pitavastatin or pravastatin undergoing percutaneous coronary intervention. *Am J Cardiol.* 2013 Jun1;111(11):1570-5.

7. Harris JI, Hibbeln JR, Mackey RH, et al. Statin treatment alters serum n-3 and n-6 fatty acids in hypercholesterolemic patients. *Prostaglandins Leukot Essent Fatty Acids.* 2004 Oct;71(4):263-9.

8. Kurisu S, Ishibashi K, Kato Y, et al. Effects of lipid-lowering therapy with strong statin on serum polyunsaturated fatty acid levels in patients with coronary artery disease. *Heart Vessels.* 2013 Jan;28(1):34-8.

9. Nozue T, Yamamoto S, Tohyama S, et al. Effects of statins on serum n-3 to n-6 polyunsaturated fatty acid ratios in patients with coronary artery disease. *Am J Cardiol.* 2013 Jan 1;111(1):6-11.

10. Morris DH. Metabolism of alpha-linolenic acid. *Flax Council of Canada*. 2014.

11. Barcelo-Coblijn G, Murphy EJ. Alpha-linolenic acid and its conversion to longer chain n-3 fatty acids: benefits for human health and a role in maintaining tissue n-3 fatty acid levels. *Prog Lipid Res*. 2009 Nov;48(6):355-74.

12. Al MD, Badart-Smook A, von Houwelingen AC, et al. Fat intake of women during normal pregnancy: relationship with maternal and neonatal essential fatty acid status. *J Am Coll Nutr*. 1996;15(1):49-55.

13. Carlson SE, Werkman SH, Peeples JM, et al. Long-chain fatty acids and early visual and cognitive development of preterm infants. *Eur J Clin Nutr*. 1994 Aug;48 Suppl 2:S27-30.

14. Hornstra G. Essential fatty acids in mothers and their neonates. *Am J Clin Nutr*. 2000 May;71(5 Suppl):1262s-9s.

15. Burdge GC, Wootton SA. Conversion of alpha-linolenic acid to eicosapentaenoic, docosapentaenoic and docosahexaenoic acids in young women. *Br J Nutr*. 2002 Oct;88:411-20.

16. Docosahexaenoic acid (DHA). Monograph. *Altern Med Rev*. 2009;14(4):391-9.

17. Hornstra G. Essential fatty acids in mothers and their neonates. *Am J Clin Nutr*. 2000 May;71(5 Suppl):1262s-9s.

18. Barcelo-Coblijn G, Murphy EJ. Alpha-linolenic acid and its conversion to longer chain n-3 fatty acids: benefits for human health and a role in maintaining tissue n-3 fatty acid levels. *Prog Lipid Res*. 2009 Nov;48(6):355-74.

19. Ibid.

20. Gibson RA, Neumann MA, Makrides M. Effect of increasing breast milk docosahexaenoic acid on plasma and erythrocyte phospholipid fatty acids and neural indices of exclusively breast fed infants. *Eur J Clin Nutr*. 1997 Sep;51(9):578-84.

21. Hornstra G. Essential fatty acids in mothers and their neonates. *Am J Clin Nutr*. 2000 May;71(5 Suppl):1262s-9s.

22. Barcelo-Coblijn G, Murphy EJ. Alpha-linolenic acid and its conversion to longer chain n-3 fatty acids: benefits for human health and a role in maintaining tissue n-3 fatty acid levels. *Prog Lipid Res*. 2009 Nov;48(6):355-74.

23. Youdim KA, Martin A, Joseph JA. Essential fatty acids and the brain: possible health implications. *Int J Dev Neurosci*. 2000 Jul-Aug;18(4-5):383-99.

24. Willatts P, Forsyth JS, DiModugno MK, et al. Effect of long-chain polyunsaturated fatty acids in infant formula on problem solving at 10 months of age. *Lancet*. 1998 Aug 29;352(9129):688-91.

25. Youdim KA, Martin A, Joseph JA. Essential fatty acids and the brain: possible health implications. *Int J Dev Neurosci*. 2000 Jul-Aug;18(4-5):383-99.

26. Barcelo-Coblijn G, Murphy EJ. Alpha-linolenic acid and its conversion to longer chain n-3 fatty acids: benefits for human health and a role in maintaining tissue n-3 fatty acid levels. *Prog Lipid Res*. 2009 Nov;48(6):355-74.

27. Lucas A, Morley R, Cole TJ, et al. Breast milk and subsequent intelligence quotient in children born preterm. *Lancet*. 1992 Feb 1;339(8788):261-4.

28. Rodgers B. Feeding in infancy and later ability and attainment: a longitudinal study. *Dev Med Child Neurol.* 1978 Aug;20(4):421-6.

29. Taylor B, Wadsworth J. Breast feeding and child development at five years. *Dev Med Child Neurol.* 1984 Feb;26(1):73-80.

30. Rogan WJ, Gladen BC. Breast-feeding and cognitive development. *Early Hum Dev.* 1993 Jan;31(3):181-93.

31. Horwood LJ, Fergusson DM. Breastfeeding and later cognitive and academic outcomes. *Pediatrics.* 1998 Jan;101(1):E9.

32. Lanting CI, Fidler V, Huisman M, et al. Neurological differences between 9-year-old children fed breast-milk or formula-milk as babies. *Lancet.* 1994 Nov 12;344(8933):1319-22.

33. Menkes JH. Early feeding history of children with learning disorders. *Dev Med Child Neurol.* 1977 Apr;19(2):169-71.

34. Rodgers B. Feeding in infancy and later ability and attainment: a longitudinal study. *Dev Med Child Neurol.* 1978 Aug;20(4):421-6.

35. Taylor B, Wadsworth J. Breast feeding and child development at five years. *Dev Med Child Neurol.* 1984 Feb;26(1):73-80.

36. Hornstra G. Essential fatty acids in mothers and their neonates. *Am J Clin Nutr.* 2000 May;71(5 Suppl):1262s-9s.

37. Popeski D, Ebbeling LR, Brown PB, et al. Blood pressure during pregnancy in Canadian Inuit: community differences related to diet. *CMAJ.* 1991 Sep 1;145(5):445-54.

38. Williams MA, Zingheim RW, King IB, et al. Omega-3 fatty acids in maternal erythrocytes and risk of preeclampsia. *Epidemiology.* 1995 May;6(3):232-7.

39. Ibid.

40. Onwude JL, Lilford RJ, Hjartardottir H, et al. A randomised double blind placebo controlled trial of fish oil in high risk pregnancy. *Br J Obstet Gynaecol.* 1995 Feb;102(2):95-100.

41. Logan AC. Neurobehavioral aspects of omega-3 fatty acids: possible mechanisms and therapeutic value in major depression. *Altern Med Rev.* 2003 Nov;8(4):410-25.

42. Klerman GL, Weissman MM. Increasing rates of depression. *JAMA.* 1989 Apr 21;261(15):2229-35.

43. Kornstein SG, Schneider RK. Clinical features of treatment-resistant depression. *J Clin Psychiatry.* 2001;62 Suppl 16:18-25.

44. Lin PY, Huang SY, Su KP. A meta-analytic review of polyunsaturated fatty acid compositions in patients with depression. *Biol Psychiatry.* 2010 Jul 15;68(2):140-7.

45. Tanskanen A, Hibbeln JR, Tuomilehto J, et al. Fish consumption and depressive symptoms in the general population in Finland. *Psychiatr Serv.* 2001 Apr;52(4):529-31.

46. Maes M, Smith RS. Fatty acids, cytokines, and major depression. *Biol Psychiatry.* 1998 Mar 1;43(5):313-4.

47. Ibid.

48. Mazereeuw G, Lanctot KL, Chau SA, et al. Effects of omega-3 fatty acids on cognitive performance: a meta-analysis. *Neurobiol Aging.* 2012 Jul;33(7):1482. e17-29.

49. Xia Z, DePierre JW, Nassberger L. Tricyclic antidepressants inhibit IL-6, IL-1 beta and TNF-alpha release in human blood monocytes and IL-2 and interferon-gamma in T cells. *Immunopharmacology.* 1996 Aug;34(1):27-37.

50. Serhan CN, Arita M, Hong S, et al. Resolvins, docosatrienes, and neuroprotectins, novel omega-3-derived mediators, and their endogenous aspirin-triggered epimers. *Lipids.* 2004 Nov;39(11):1125-32.

51. Hibbeln JR. Fish consumption and major depression. *Lancet.* 1998 Apr 18;351(9110):1213.

52. Hibbeln JR, Gow RV. The potential for military diets to reduce depression, suicide, and impulsive aggression: a review of current evidence for omega-3 and omega-6 fatty acids. *Mil Med.* 2014 Nov;17911 Suppl):117-28.

53. Tanskanen A, Hibbeln JR, Tuomilehto J, et al. Fish consumption and depressive symptoms in the general population in Finland. *Psychiatr Serv.* 2001 Apr;52(4):529-31.

54. Silvers KM, Scott KM. Fish consumption and self-reported physical and mental health status. *Public Health Nutr.* 2002 Jun;5(3):427-31.

55. Adams PB, Lawson S, Sanigorski A, et al. Arachidonic acid to eicosapentaenoic acid ratio in blood correlates positively with clinical symptoms of depression. *Lipids.* 1996 Mar;31 Suppl:S157-61.

56. Tiemeier H, van Tuijl HR, Hofman A, et al. Plasma fatty acid composition and depression are associated in the elderly: the Rotterdam Study. *Am J Clin Nutr.* 2003 Jul;78(1):40-6.

57. Mamalakis G, Tornaritis M, Kafatos A. Depression and adipose essential polyunsaturated fatty acids. *Prostaglandins Leukot Essent Fatty Acids.* 2002 Nov;67(5):311-8.

58. Hibbeln JR. Seafood consumption, the DHA content of mothers' milk and prevalence rates of postpartum depression: a cross-national, ecological analysis. *J Affect Disord.* 2002 May;69(1-3):15-29.

59. Mazereeuw G, Lanctot KL, Chau SA, et al. Effects of omega-3 fatty acids on cognitive performance: a meta-analysis. *Neurobiol Aging.* 2012 Jul;33(7):1482. e17-29.

60. Ibid.

61. Ibid.

62. Nemets B, Stahl Z, Belmaker RH. Addition of omega-3 fatty acid to maintenance medication treatment for recurrent unipolar depressive disorder. *Am J Psychiatry.* 2002 Mar;159(3):477-9.

63. Su KP, Huang SY, Chiu CC, et al. Omega-3 fatty acids in major depressive disorder. A preliminary double-blind, placebo-controlled trial. *Eur Neuropsychopharmacol.* 2003 Aug;13(4):267-71.

64. Lin PY, Huang SY, Su KP. A meta-analytic review of polyunsaturated fatty acid compositions in patients with depression. *Biol Psychiatry.* 2010 Jul 15;68(2):140-7.

65. Grosso G, Pajak A, Marventano S, et al. Role of omega-3 fatty acids in the treatment of depressive disorders: a comprehensive meta-analysis of randomized clinical trials. *PLoS One.* 2014;9(5):e96905.

66. Nemets B, Stahl Z, Belmaker RH. Addition of omega-3 fatty acid to maintenance medication treatment for recurrent unipolar depressive disorder. *Am J Psychiatry.* 2002 Mar;159(3):477-9.

67. Peet M, Horrobin DF. A dose-ranging study of the effects of ethyl-eicosapentaenoate in patients with ongoing depression despite apparently adequate treatment with standard drugs. *Arch Gen Psychiatry.* 2002 Oct;59(1):913-9.

68. Frangou S, Lewis M, McCrone P. Efficacy of ethyl-eicosapentaenoic acid in bipolar depression: randomised double-blind placebo-controlled study. *Br J Psychiatry.* 2006 Jan;188:46-50.

69. Nemets H, Nemets B, Apter A, et al. Omega-3 treatment of childhood depression: a controlled, double-blind pilot study. *Am J Psychiatry.* 2006 Jun;163(6):1098-100.

70. Su KP, Huang SY, Chiu TH, et al. Omega-3 fatty acids for major depressive disorder during pregnancy: results from a randomized, double-blind, placebo-controlled trial. *J Clin Psychiatry.* 2008 Apr;69(4):644-51.

71. Jazayeri S, Tehrani-Doost M, Keshavarz SA, et al. Comparison of therapeutic effects of omega-3 fatty acid eicosapentaenoic acid and fluoxetine, separately and in combination, in major depressive disorder. *Aust N Z J Psychiatry.* 2008 Mar;42(3):192-8.

72. Jadoon A, Chiu CC, McDermott L, et al. Associations of polyunsaturated fatty acids with residual depression or anxiety in older people with major depression. *J Affect Disord.* 2012 Feb;136(3):918-25.

73. Wolfe AR, Ogbonna EM, Lim S, et al. Dietary linoleic and oleic fatty acids in relation to severe depressed mood: 10 years follow-up of a national cohort. *Prog Neuropsychopharmacol Biol Psychiatry.* 2009 Aug 31;33(6):972-7.

74. Lucas M, Mirzaei F, O'Reilly EJ, et al. Dietary intake of n-3 and n-6 fatty acids and the risk of clinical depression in women: a 10-y prospective follow-up study. *Am J Clin Nutr.* 2011 Jun;93(6):1337-43.

75. Kidd PM. Omega-3 DHA and EPA for cognition, behavior, and mood: clinical findings and structural-functional synergies with cell membrane phospholipids. *Altern Med Rev.* 2007 Sep;12(3):207-27.

76. Ibid.

77. Hirayama S, Hamazaki T, Terasawa K. Effect of docosahexaenoic acid-containing food administration on symptoms of attention-deficit/hyperactivity disorder - a placebo-controlled double-blind study. *Eur J Clin Nutr.* 2004 Mar;58(3):467-73.

78. Stevens L, Zhang W, Peck L, et al. EFA supplementation in children with inattention, hyperactivity, and other disruptive behaviors. *Lipids.* 2003 Oct;38(1):1007-21.

79. Vancassel S, Durand G, Barthelemy C, et al. Plasma fatty acid levels in autistic children. *Prostaglandins Leukot Essent Fatty Acids.* 2001 Jul;65(1):1-7.

80. Kidd PM. Omega-3 DHA and EPA for cognition, behavior, and mood: clinical findings and structural-functional synergies with cell membrane phospholipids. *Altern Med Rev.* 2007 Sep;12(3):207-27.

81. Ibid.

82. Amminger GP, Berger GE, Schafer MR, et al. Omega-3 fatty acids supplementation in children with autism: a double-blind randomized, placebo-controlled pilot study. *Biol Psychiatry.* 2007 Feb 15;61(4):551-3.

83. Kidd PM. Omega-3 DHA and EPA for cognition, behavior, and mood: clinical findings and structural-functional synergies with cell membrane phospholipids. *Altern Med Rev.* 2007 Sep;12(3):207-27.

84. Fontani G, Corradeschi F, Felici A, et al. Cognitive and physiological effects of omega-3 polyunsaturated fatty acid supplementation in healthy subjects. *Eur J Clin Invest.* 2005 Nov;35(11):691-9.

85. Kidd PM. Omega-3 DHA and EPA for cognition, behavior, and mood: clinical findings and structural-functional synergies with cell membrane phospholipids. *Altern Med Rev.* 2007 Sep;12(3):207-27.

86. Zanarini MC, Frankenburg FR. Omega-3 fatty acid treatment of women with borderline personality disorder: a double-blind, placebo-controlled pilot study. *Am J Psychiatry.* 2003 Jan;160(1):167-9.

87. De Vriese SR, Christophe AB, Maes M. In humans, the seasonal variation in poly-unsaturated fatty acids is related to the seasonal variation in violent suicide and serotonergic markers of violent suicide. *Prostaglandins Leukot Essent Fatty Acids.* 2004 Jul;71(1):13-8.

88. Lewis MD, Hibbeln JR, Johnson JE, et al. Suicide deaths of active-duty US military and omega-3 fatty-acid status: a case-control comparison. *J Clin Psychiatry.* 2011 Dec;72(1):1585-90.

89. Huan M, Hamazaki K, Sun Y, et al. Suicide attempt and n-3 fatty acid levels in red blood cells: a case control study in China. *Biol Psychiatry.* 2004 Oct 1;56(7):490-6.

90. Hallahan B, Hibbeln JR, Davis JM, et al. Omega-3 fatty acid supplementation in patients with recurrent self-harm. Single-centre double-blind randomised controlled trial. *Br J Psychiatry.* 2007 Feb;190:118-22.

91. Green P, Hermesh H, Monselise A, et al. Red cell membrane omega-3 fatty acids are decreased in nondepressed patients with social anxiety disorder. *Eur Neuropsychopharmacol.* 2006 Feb;16(2):107-13.

92. Chiu CC, Huang SY, Su KP, et al. Polyunsaturated fatty acid deficit in patients with bipolar mania. *Eur Neuropsychopharmacol.* 2003 Mar;13(2):99-103.

93. Kidd PM. Omega-3 DHA and EPA for cognition, behavior, and mood: clinical findings and structural-functional synergies with cell membrane phospholipids. *Altern Med Rev.* 2007 Sep;12(3):207-27.

94. Connor WE, Connor SL. The importance of fish and docosahexaenoic acid in Alzheimer disease. *Am J Clin Nutr.* 2007 Apr;85(4):929-30.

95. Andlin-Sobocki P, Jonsson B, Wittchen HU, et al. Cost of disorders of the brain in Europe. *Eur J Neurol.* 2005 Jun;12 Suppl 1:1-27.

96. Olesen J, Gustavsson A, Svensson M, et al. The economic cost of brain disorders in Europe. *Eur J Neurol.* 2012 Jan;19(1):155-62.

97. Prasad MR, Lovell MA, Yatin M, et al. Regional membrane phospholipid alterations in Alzheimer's disease. *Neurochem Res.* 1998 Jan;23(1):81-8.

98. Kidd PM. Omega-3 DHA and EPA for cognition, behavior, and mood: clinical findings and structural-functional synergies with cell membrane phospholipids. *Altern Med Rev.* 2007 Sep;12(3):207-27.

99. Das UN. Essential fatty acids: biochemistry, physiology and pathology. *Biotechnology J.* 2006 Apr;1(4):420-39.

100. Moyad MA. An introduction to dietary/supplemental omega-3 fatty acids for general health and prevention: part II. *Urol Oncol.* 2005 Jan-Feb;23(1):36-48.

101. Kalmijn S, Launer LJ, Ott A, et al. Dietary fat intake and the risk of incident dementia in the Rotterdam Study. *Ann Neurol.* 1997 Nov;42(5):776-82.

102. Barberger-Gateau P, Letenneur L, Deschamps V, et al. Fish, meat, and risk of dementia: cohort study. *BMJ.* 2002 Oct 26;325(7370):932-3.

103. Morris MC, Evans DA, Bienias JL, et al. Consumption of fish and n-3 fatty acids and risk of incident Alzheimer disease. *Arch Neurol.* 2003 Jul;60(7):940-6.

104. Freemantle E, Vandal M, Tremblay-Mercier J, et al. Omega-3 fatty acids, energy substrates, and brain function during aging. *Prostaglandins Leukot Essent Fatty Acids.* 2006 Sep;75(3):213-20.

105. Ibid.

106. Ibid.

107. Ibid.

108. Ibid.

109. Tully AM, Roche HM, Doyle R, et al. Low serum cholesteryl ester-docosahexaenoic acid levels in Alzheimer's disease: a case-control study. *Br J Nutr.* 2003 Apr;89(4):483-9.

110. Conquer JA, Tierney MC, Zecevic J, et al. Fatty acid analysis of blood plasma of patients with Alzheimer's disease, other types of dementia, and cognitive impairment. *Lipids.* 2000 Dec;35(12):1305-12.

111. Huang TL. Omega-3 fatty acids, cognitive decline, and Alzheimer's disease: a critical review and evaluation of the literature. *J Alzheimers Dis.* 2010;21(3):673-90.

112. Whalley LJ, Deary IJ, Starr JM, et al. n-3 Fatty acid erythrocyte membrane content, APOE varepsilon4, and cognitive variation: an observational follow-up study in late adulthood. *Am J Clin Nutr.* 2008 Feb;87(2):449-54.

113. Mazereeuw G, Lanctot KL, Chau SA, et al. Effects of omega-3 fatty acids on cognitive performance: a meta-analysis. *Neurobiol Aging.* 2012 Jul;33(7):1482. e17-29.

114. Freemantle E, Vandal M, Tremblay-Mercier J, et al. Omega-3 fatty acids, energy substrates, and brain function during aging. *Prostaglandins Leukot Essent Fatty Acids.* 2006 Sep;75(3):213-20.

115. Conquer JA, Tierney MC, Zecevic J, et al. Fatty acid analysis of blood plasma of patients with Alzheimer's disease, other types of dementia, and cognitive impairment. *Lipids.* 2000 Dec;35(12):1305-12.

116. Schaefer EJ, Bongard V, Beiser AS, et al. Plasma phosphatidylcholine docosahexaenoic acid content and risk of dementia and Alzheimer disease: the Framingham Heart Study. *Arch Neurol.* 2006 Nov;63(11):1545-50.

117. Freund-Levi Y, Eriksdotter-Jonhagen M, Cederholm T, et al. Omega-3 fatty acid treatment in 174 patients with mild to moderate Alzheimer disease: OmegAD study: a randomized double-blind trial. *Arch Neurol.* 2006 Oct;63(1):1402-8.

118. Mazereeuw G, Lanctot KL, Chau SA, et al. Effects of omega-3 fatty acids on cognitive performance: a meta-analysis. *Neurobiol Aging.* 2012 Jul;33(7):1482. e17-29.

119. Shinto L, Quinn J, Montine T, et al. A randomized placebo-controlled pilot trial of omega-3 fatty acids and alpha lipoic acid in Alzheimer's disease. *J Alzheimers Dis.* 2014;38(1):111-20.

120. Mazereeuw G, Lanctot KL, Chau SA, et al. Effects of omega-3 fatty acids on cognitive performance: a meta-analysis. *Neurobiol Aging.* 2012 Jul;33(7):1482. e17-29.

121. Kalmijn S, Launer LJ, Ott A, et al. Dietary fat intake and the risk of incident dementia in the Rotterdam Study. *Ann Neurol.* 1997 Nov;42(5):776-82.

122. Barberger-Gateau P, Letenneur L, Deschamps V, et al. Fish, meat, and risk of dementia: cohort study. *BMJ.* 2002 Oct 26;325(7370):932-3.

123. Richardson AJ, Puri BK. A randomized double-blind, placebo-controlled study of the effects of supplementation with highly unsaturated fatty acids on ADHD-related symptoms in children with specific learning difficulties. *Prog Neuropsychopharmacol Biol Psychiatry.* 2002 Feb;26(2):233-9.

124. Vancassel S, Durand G, Barthelemy C, et al. Plasma fatty acid levels in autistic children. *Prostaglandins Leukot Essent Fatty Acids.* 2001 Jul;65(1):1-7.

125. Mamalakis G, Tornaritis M, Kafatos A. Depression and adipose essential polyunsaturated fatty acids. *Prostaglandins Leukot Essent Fatty Acids.* 2002 Nov;67(5):311-8.

126. Mamalakis G, Kalogeropoulos N, Andrikopoulos N, et al. Depression and long chain n-3 fatty acids in adipose tissue in adults from Crete. *Eur J Clin Nutr.* 2006 Jul;60(7):882-8.

127. Zanarini MC, Frankenburg FR. Omega-3 fatty acid treatment of women with borderline personality disorder: a double-blind, placebo-controlled pilot study. *Am J Psychiatry.* 2003 Jan;160(1):167-9.

128. Assies J, Lieverse R, Vreken P, et al. Significantly reduced docosahexaenoic and docosapentaenoic acid concentrations in erythrocyte membranes from schizophrenic patients compared with a carefully matched control group. *Biol Psychiatry.* 2001 Mar 15;49(6):510-22.

129. Hamazaki T, Sawazaki S, Itomura M, et al. Effect of docosahexaenoic acid on hostility. *World Rev Nutr Diet.* 2001;88:47-52.

130. Mamalakis G, Kafatos A, Tornaritis M, et al. Anxiety and adipose essential fatty acid precursors for prostaglandin E1 and E2. *J Am Coll Nutr.* 1998 Jun;17(3):239-43.

131. Shakeri J, Khanegi M, Golshani S, et al. Effects of omega-3 supplement in the treatment of patients with bipolar I disorder. *Int J Prev Med.* 2016 May 19;7:77.

132. Vesco AT, Lehmann J, Gracious BL, et al. Omega-3 supplementation for psychotic mania and comorbid anxiety in children. *J Child Adolesc Psychopharmacol.* 2015 Sep 1;25(7):526-34.

133. Cott J, Hibbeln JR. Lack of seasonal mood change in Icelanders. *Am J Psychiatry.* 2001 Feb;158(2):328.

134. Wong-Ekkabut J, Xu Z, Triampo W, et al. Effect of lipid peroxidation on the properties of lipid bilayers: a molecular dynamics study. *Biophys J.* 2007 Dec 15;93(12):4225-36.

135. Spiteller G. Peroxyl radicals: inductors of neurodegenerative and other inflammatory diseases. Their origin and how they transform cholesterol, phospholipids, plasmalogens, polyunsaturated fatty acids, sugars, and proteins into deleterious products. *Free Radic Biol Med.* 2006 Aug 1;41(3):362-87.

136. Ibid.

137. Ibid.

138. Moran JH, Mon T, Hendrickson TL, et al. Defining mechanisms of toxicity for linoleic acid monoepoxides and diols in Sf-21 cells. *Chem Res Toxicol.* 2001 Apr;14(4):431-7.

139. Montine TJ, Amarnath V, Martin ME, et al. E-4-hydroxy-2-nonenal is cytotoxic and cross-links cytoskeletal proteins in P19 neuroglial cultures. *Am J Pathol.* 1996 Jan;148(1):89-93.

140. Best KP, Gold M, Kennedy D, et al. Omega-3 long-chain PUFA intake during pregnancy and allergic disease outcomes in the offspring: a systematic review and meta-analysis of observational studies and randomized controlled trials. *Am J Clin Nutr.* 2016 Jan;103(1):128-43.

141. Ibid.

142. Ibid.

143. Maslova E, Strom M, Oken E, et al. Fish intake during pregnancy and the risk of child asthma and allergic rhinitis - longitudinal evidence from the Danish National Birth Cohort. *Br J Nutr.* 2013 Oct;110(7):1313-25.

144. Nwaru BI, Erkkola M, Lumia M, et al. Maternal intake of fatty acids during pregnancy and allergies in the offspring. *Br J Nutr.* 2012 Aug;108(4):720-32.

145. Jedrychowski W, Perera F, Maugeri U, et al. Effects of prenatal and perinatal exposure to fine air pollutants and maternal fish consumption on the occurrence of infantile eczema. *Int Arch Allergy Immunol.* 2011;155(3):275-81.

146. Willers SM, Devereux G, Craig LC, et al. Maternal food consumption during pregnancy and asthma, respiratory and atopic symptoms in 5-year-old children. *Thorax.* 2007 Sep;62(9):773-9.

147. Janakiram NB, Mohammed A, Rao CV. Role of lipoxins, resolvins, and other bioactive lipids in colon and pancreatic cancer. *Cancer Metastasis Rev.* 2011 Dec;30(3-4):507-23.

148. Gonzalez MJ, Schemmel RA, Gray JI, et al. Effect of dietary fat on growth of MCF-7 and MDA-MB231 human breast carcinomas in athymic nude mice: relationship between carcinoma growth and lipid peroxidation product levels. *Carcinogenesis.* 1991 Jul;12(7):1231-5.

149. Gonzalez MJ, Schemmel RA, Dugan L, Jr., et al. Dietary fish oil inhibits human breast carcinoma growth: a function of increased lipid peroxidation. *Lipids.* 1993 Sep;28(9):827-32.

150. Hudson EA, Beck SA, Tisdale MJ. Kinetics of the inhibition of tumour growth in mice by eicosapentaenoic acid-reversal by linoleic acid. *Biochem Pharmacol.* 1993 Jun 9;45(11):2189-94.

151. Conklin KA. Dietary polyunsaturated fatty acids: impact on cancer chemotherapy and radiation. *Altern Med Rev.* 2002 Feb;7(1):4-21.

152. Ibid.

153. Ibid.

154. Ibid.

Chapter 7

1. Ogden CL, Carroll MD, Kit BK, et al. Prevalence of obesity in the United States, 2009-2010. *NCHS data brief.* 2012 Jan:(82)1-8.

2. Yki-Jarvinen H. Fat in the liver and insulin resistance. *Ann Med.* 2005;37(5): 347-56.

3. Jung SH, Ha KH, Kim DJ. Visceral fat mass has stronger associations with diabetes and prediabetes than other anthropometric obesity indicators among Korean adults. *Yonsei Med J.* 2016 May 1;57(3):674-80.

4. Sheth SG, Chopra Sanjive. Epidemiology, clinical features, and diagnosis of nonalcoholic fatty liver disease in adults [Internet]. *UpToDate.* 2018. Available from http://www.uptodate.com/contents/epidemiology-clinical-features-and -diagnosis-of-nonalcoholic-fatty-liver-disease-in-adults.

5. Vernon G, Baranova A, Younossi ZM. Systematic review: the epidemiology and natural history of non-alcoholic fatty liver disease and non-alcoholic steatohepatitis in adults. *Aliment Pharmacol Ther.* 2011 Aug;34(3):274-85.

6. Williams CD, Stengel J, Asike MI, et al. Prevalence of nonalcoholic fatty liver disease and nonalcoholic steatohepatitis among a largely middle-aged population utilizing ultrasound and liver biopsy: a prospective study. *Gastroenterology.* 2011 Jan;140(1):124-31.

7. Menke A, Casagrande S, Geiss L, et al. Prevalence of and trends in diabetes among adults in the United States, 1988-2012. *JAMA.* 2015 Sep 8;314(1):1021-9.

8. Lopategi A, Lopez-Vicario C, Alcaraz-Quiles J, et al. Role of bioactive lipid mediators in obese adipose tissue inflammation and endocrine dysfunction. *Mol Cell Endocrinol.* 2016 Jan5;419:44-59.

9. Ibid.

10. Claria J, Nguyen BT, Madenci AL, et al. Diversity of lipid mediators in human adipose tissue depots. *Am J Physiol Cell Physiol.* 2013 Jun 15;304(12):C1141-9.

11. Claria J, Dalli J, Yacoubian S, et al. Resolvin D1 and resolvin D2 govern local inflammatory tone in obese fat. *J Immunol.* 2012 Sep 1;189(5):2597-605.

12. Lopategi A, Lopez-Vicario C, Alcaraz-Quiles J, et al. Role of bioactive lipid mediators in obese adipose tissue inflammation and endocrine dysfunction. *Mol Cell Endocrinol.* 2016 Jan5;419:44-59.

13. White PJ, Arita M, Taguchi R, et al. Transgenic restoration of long-chain n-3 fatty acids in insulin target tissues improves resolution capacity and alleviates obesity-linked inflammation and insulin resistance in high-fat-fed mice. *Diabetes.* 2010 Dec;59(12):3066-73.

14. Neuhofer A, Zeyda M, Mascher D, et al. Impaired local production of proresolving lipid mediators in obesity and 17-HDHA as a potential treatment for obesity-associated inflammation. *Diabetes.* 2013 Jun;62(6):1945-56.

15. Hellmann J, Tang Y, Kosuri M, et al. Resolvin D1 decreases adipose tissue macrophage accumulation and improves insulin sensitivity in obese-diabetic mice. *FASEB J.* 2011 Jul;25(7):2399-407.

16. Lopategi A, Lopez-Vicario C, Alcaraz-Quiles J, et al. Role of bioactive lipid mediators in obese adipose tissue inflammation and endocrine dysfunction. *Mol Cell Endocrinol.* 2016 Jan5;419:44-59.

17. Ibid.

18. Guyenet SJ, Carlson SE. Increase in adipose tissue linoleic acid of US adults in the last half century. *Advances in Nutrition.* 2015 Nov 1;6(6):660-4.

19. Surette ME, Koumenis IL, Edens MB, et al. Inhibition of leukotriene synthesis, pharmacokinetics, and tolerability of a novel dietary fatty acid formulation in healthy adult subjects. *Clin Ther.* 2003 Mar;25(3):948-71.

20. James MJ, Gibson RA, Cleland LG. Dietary polyunsaturated fatty acids and inflammatory mediator production. *Am J Clin Nutr.* 2000 Jan;71(1 Suppl):343s-8s.

21. Manole, Bogdan A. Effect of alpha-linolenic acid on global fatty oxidation in adipocytes and skeletal muscle cells [honors thesis project]. University of Tennessee; 2011.

22. Ikemoto S, Takahashi M, Tsunoda N, et al. High-fat diet-induced hyperglycemia and obesity in mice: differential effects of dietary oils. *Metabolism.* 1996 Dec;45(12):1539-46.

23. Hill JO, Peters JC, Lin D, et al. Lipid accumulation and body fat distribution is influenced by type of dietary fat fed to rats. *Int J Obes Relat Metab Disord.* 1993 Apr;17(4):223-36.

24. Flachs P, Rossmeisl M, Kuda O, et al. Stimulation of mitochondrial oxidative capacity in white fat independent of UCP1: a key to lean phenotype. *Biochim Biophys Acta.* 2013 May;1831(5):986-1003.

25. Flachs P, Horakova O, Brauner P, et al. Polyunsaturated fatty acids of marine origin upregulate mitochondrial biogenesis and induce beta-oxidation in white fat. *Diabetologia*. 2005 Nov;48(11):2365-75.

26. Hensler M, Bardova K, Jilkova ZM, et al. The inhibition of fat cell proliferation by n-3 fatty acids in dietary obese mice. *Lipids Health Dis*. 2011 Aug 2;10:128.

27. Ruzickova J, Rossmeisl M, Prazak T, et al. Omega-3 PUFA of marine origin limit diet-induced obesity in mice by reducing cellularity of adipose tissue. *Lipids*. 2004 Dec;39(12):1177-85.

28. Spalding KL, Arner E, Westermark PO, et al. Dynamics of fat cell turnover in humans. *Nature*. 2008 Jun 5;453(7196):783-7.

29. Azain MJ. Role of fatty acids in adipocyte growth and development. *J Anim Sci*. 2004 Mar;82(3):916-24.

30. Hutley LJ, Newell FM, Joyner JM, et al. Effects of rosiglitazone and linoleic acid on human preadipocyte differentiation. *Eur J Clin Invest*. 2003 Jul;33(7):574-81.

31. Alvheim AR, Malde MK, Osei-Hyiaman D, et al. Dietary linoleic acid elevates endogenous 2-AG and anandamide and induces obesity. *Obesity (Silver Spring)*. 2012 Oct;20(1):1984-94.

32. Massiera F, Saint-Marc P, Seydoux J, et al. Arachidonic acid and prostacyclin signaling promote adipose tissue development: a human health concern? *J Lipid Res*. 2003 Feb;44(2):271-9.

33. Moon RJ, Harvey NC, Robinson SM, et al. Maternal plasma polyunsaturated fatty acid status in late pregnancy is associated with offspring body composition in childhood. *J Clin Endocrinol Metab*. 2013 Jan;98(1):299-307.

34. Donahue SM, Rifas-Shiman SL, Gold DR, et al. Prenatal fatty acid status and child adiposity at age 3 y: results from a US pregnancy cohort. *Am J Clin Nutr*. 2011 Apr;93(4):780-8.

35. Hill JO, Peters JC, Lin D, et al. Lipid accumulation and body fat distribution is influenced by type of dietary fat fed to rats. *Int J Obes Relat Metab Disord*. 1993 Apr;17(4):223-36.

36. Su W, Jones PJ. Dietary fatty acid composition influences energy accretion in rats. *J Nutr*. 1993 Dec;123(12):2109-14.

37. Baillie RA, Takada R, Nakamura M, et al. Coordinate induction of peroxisomal acyl-CoA oxidase and UCP-3 by dietary fish oil: a mechanism for decreased body fat deposition. *Prostaglandins Leukot Essent Fatty Acids*. 1999 May-Jun;60(5-6):351-6.

38. Belzung F, Raclot T, Groscolas R. Fish oil n-3 fatty acids selectively limit the hypertrophy of abdominal fat depots in growing rats fed high-fat diets. *Am J Physiol*. 1993 Jun;264(6 Pt 2):R1111-8.

39. Kunesova M, Braunerova R, Hlavaty P, et al. The influence of n-3 polyunsaturated fatty acids and very low calorie diet during a short-term weight reducing regimen on weight loss and serum fatty acid composition in severely obese women. *Physiol Res*. 2006;55(1):63-72.

40. Ibid.

41. Thorsdottir I, Tomasson H, Gunnarsdottir I, et al. Randomized trial of weight-loss-diets for young adults varying in fish and fish oil content. *Int J Obes (Lond).* 2007 Oct;31(1):1560-6.

42. Mater MK, Thelen AP, Pan DA, et al. Sterol response element-binding protein 1c (SREBP1c) is involved in the polyunsaturated fatty acid suppression of hepatic S14 gene transcription. *J Biol Chem.* 1999 Nov;274(46):32725-32.

43. Hulbert AJ, Else PL. Membranes as possible pacemakers of metabolism. *J Theor Biol.* 1999 Aug 7;199(3):257-74.

44. Allport S. The queen of fats: why omega-3s were removed from the western diet and what we can do to replace them. Oakland (CA): University of California Press; 2006. 232 p.

45. Hulbert AJ, Else PL. Membranes as possible pacemakers of metabolism. *J Theor Biol.* 1999 Aug 7;199(3):257-74.

46. Ibid.

47. Smith GI, Atherton P, Reeds DN, et al. Dietary omega-3 fatty acid supplementation increases the rate of muscle protein synthesis in older adults: a randomized controlled trial. *Am J Clin Nutr.* 2011 Feb;93(2):402-12.

48. Smith GI, Julliand S, Reeds DN, et al. Fish oil-derived n-3 PUFA therapy increases muscle mass and function in healthy older adults. *Am J Clin Nutr.* 2015 Jul;102(1):115-22.

49. Gingras AA, White PJ, Chouinard PY, et al. Long-chain omega-3 fatty acids regulate bovine whole-body protein metabolism by promoting muscle insulin signalling to the Akt-mTOR-S6K1 pathway and insulin sensitivity. *J Physiol.* 2007 Feb 15;579(Pt 1):269-84.

50. Alexander JW, Saito H, Trocki O, et al. The importance of lipid type in the diet after burn injury. *Ann Surg.* 1986 Jul;204(1):1-8.

51. Berbert AA, Kondo CR, Almendra CL, et al. Supplementation of fish oil and olive oil in patients with rheumatoid arthritis. *Nutrition.* 2005 Feb;21(2):131-6.

52. Murphy RA, Mourtzakis M, Chu QS, et al. Nutritional intervention with fish oil provides a benefit over standard of care for weight and skeletal muscle mass in patients with nonsmall cell lung cancer receiving chemotherapy. *Cancer.* 2011 Apr 15;117(8):1775-82.

53. Rodacki CL, Rodacki AL, Pereira G, et al. Fish-oil supplementation enhances the effects of strength training in elderly women. *Am J Clin Nutr.* 2012 Feb;95(2):428-36.

54. Ryan AM, Reynolds JV, Healy L, et al. Enteral nutrition enriched with eicosapentaenoic acid (EPA) preserves lean body mass following esophageal cancer surgery: results of a double-blinded randomized controlled trial. *Ann Surg.* 2009 Mar;249(3):355-63.

55. Whitehouse AS, Smith HJ, Drake JL, et al. Mechanism of attenuation of skeletal muscle protein catabolism in cancer cachexia by eicosapentaenoic acid. *Cancer Res.* 2001 May;61(9):3604-9.

56. Smith GI, Julliand S, Reeds DN, et al. Fish oil-derived n-3 PUFA therapy increases muscle mass and function in healthy older adults. *Am J Clin Nutr.* 2015 Jul;102(1):115-22.

57. Jucker BM, Cline GW, Barucci N, et al. Differential effects of safflower oil versus fish oil feeding on insulin-stimulated glycogen synthesis, glycolysis, and pyruvate dehydrogenase flux in skeletal muscle: a 13C nuclear magnetic resonance study. *Diabetes.* 1999 Jan;48(1):134-40.

58. Neschen S, Moore I, Regittnig W, et al. Contrasting effects of fish oil and safflower oil on hepatic peroxisomal and tissue lipid content. *Am J Physiol Endocrinol Metab.* 2002 Feb;282(2):E395-401.

59. Vaughan RA, Garcia-Smith R, Bisoffi M, et al. Conjugated linoleic acid or omega 3 fatty acids increase mitochondrial biosynthesis and metabolism in skeletal muscle cells. *Lipids Health Dis.* 2012 Oct 30;11:142.

60. Rodacki CL, Rodacki AL, Pereira G, et al. Fish-oil supplementation enhances the effects of strength training in elderly women. *Am J Clin Nutr.* 2012 Feb;95(2):428-36.

61. Peoples GE, McLennan PL, Howe PR, et al. Fish oil reduces heart rate and oxygen consumption during exercise. *J Cardiovasc Pharmacol.* 2008 Dec;52(6):540-7.

Chapter 8

1. Van Woudenbergh GJ, Kuijsten A, Van der Kallen CJ, et al. Comparison of fatty acid proportions in serum cholesteryl esters among people with different glucose tolerance status: the CoDAM study. *Nutr Metab Cardiovasc Dis.* 2012 Feb;22(2):133-40.

2. Adapted from Eicosanoids [Internet]. *Wikipedia.* Available from https://upload .wikimedia.org/wikipedia/commons/5/58/EFA_to_Eicosanoids.svg.

3. Van Woudenbergh GJ, Kuijsten A, Van der Kallen CJ, et al. Comparison of fatty acid proportions in serum cholesteryl esters among people with different glucose tolerance status: the CoDAM study. *Nutr Metab Cardiovasc Dis.* 2012 Feb;22(2):133-40.

4. Salomaa V, Ahola I, Tuomilehto J, et al. Fatty acid composition of serum cholesterol esters in different degrees of glucose intolerance: a population-based study. *Metabolism.* 1990 Dec;39(1):1285-91.

5. Steffen LM, Vessby B, Jacobs DR, Jr., et al. Serum phospholipid and cholesteryl ester fatty acids and estimated desaturase activities are related to overweight and cardiovascular risk factors in adolescents. *Int J Obes (Lond).* 2008 Aug;32(8):1297-304.

6. Warensjo E, Rosell M, Hellenius ML, et al. Associations between estimated fatty acid desaturase activities in serum lipids and adipose tissue in humans: links to obesity and insulin resistance. *Lipids Health Dis.* 2009 Aug 27;8:37.

7. Pan DA, Lillioja S, Milner MR, et al. Skeletal muscle membrane lipid composition is related to adiposity and insulin action. *J Clin Invest.* 1995 Dec;96(6):2802-8.

8. Brenner RR. Hormonal modulation of delta6 and delta5 desaturases: case of diabetes. *Prostaglandins Leukot Essent Fatty Acids.* 2003 Feb;68(2):151-62.

9. Ibid.

10. Bezard J, Blond JP, Bernard A, et al. The metabolism and availability of essential fatty acids in animal and human tissues. *Reprod Nutr Dev.* 1994;34(6):539-68.

11. Emken EA, Adlof RO, Gulley RM. Dietary linoleic acid influences desaturation and acylation of deuterium-labeled linoleic and linolenic acids in young adult males. *Biochim Biophys Acta.* 1994 Aug 4;1213(3):277-88.

12. St-Onge MP, Bosarge A, Goree LL, et al. Medium chain triglyceride oil consumption as part of a weight loss diet does not lead to an adverse metabolic profile when compared to olive oil. *J Am Coll Nutr.* 2008 Oct;27(5):547-52.

13. Van Wymelbeke V, Himaya A, Louis-Sylvestre J, et al. Influence of medium-chain and long-chain triacylglycerols on the control of food intake in men. *Am J Clin Nutr.* 1998 Aug;68(2):226-34.

14. Mumme K, Stonehouse W. Effects of medium-chain triglycerides on weight loss and body composition: a meta-analysis of randomized controlled trials. *J Acad Nutr Diet.* 2015 Feb;115(2):249-63.

15. Binnert C, Pachiaudi C, Beylot M, et al. Influence of human obesity on the metabolic fate of dietary long- and medium-chain triacylglycerols. *Am J Clin Nutr.* 1998 Apr;67(4):595-601.

16. Assuncao ML, Ferreira HS, dos Santos AF, et al. Effects of dietary coconut oil on the biochemical and anthropometric profiles of women presenting abdominal obesity. *Lipids.* 2009 Jul;44(7):593-601.

17. Liau KM, Lee YY, Chen CK, et al. An open-label pilot study to assess the efficacy and safety of virgin coconut oil in reducing visceral adiposity. *ISRN Pharmacol.* 2011;2011:949686.

18. DeLany JP, Windhauser MM, Champagne CM, et al. Differential oxidation of individual dietary fatty acids in humans. *Am J Clin Nutr.* 2000 Oct;72(4):905-11.

19. Lasekan JB, Rivera J, Hirvonen MD, et al. Energy expenditure in rats maintained with intravenous or intragastric infusion of total parenteral nutrition solutions containing medium- or long-chain triglyceride emulsions. *J Nutr.* 1992 Jul;122(7):1483-92.

20. DeLany JP, Windhauser MM, Champagne CM, et al. Differential oxidation of individual dietary fatty acids in humans. *Am J Clin Nutr.* 2000 Oct;72(4):905-11.

21. Ibid.

22. Leyton J, Drury PJ, Crawford MA. Differential oxidation of saturated and unsaturated fatty acids in vivo in the rat. *Br J Nutr.* 1987 May;57(3):383-93.

23. Lasekan JB, Rivera J, Hirvonen MD, et al. Energy expenditure in rats maintained with intravenous or intragastric infusion of total parenteral nutrition solutions containing medium- or long-chain triglyceride emulsions. *J Nutr.* 1992 Jul;122(7):1483-92.

24. McCarty MF, DiNicolantonio JJ. Lauric acid-rich medium-chain triglycerides can substitute for other oils in cooking applications and may have limited pathogenicity. *Open Heart.* 2016 Jul 27;3(2):105.

25. Albert BB, Derraik JG, Cameron-Smith D, et al. Fish oil supplements in New Zealand are highly oxidised and do not meet label content of n-3 PUFA. *Sci Rep* 2015;5:7928.

26. von Schacky C. Cardiovascular disease prevention and treatment. *Prostaglandins Leukot Essent Fatty Acids.* 2009 Aug-Sep;81(2-3):193-8.

27. Bunea R, El Farrah K, Deutsch L. Evaluation of the effects of Neptune Krill Oil on the clinical course of hyperlipidemia. *Altern Med Rev.* 2004 Dec;9(4):420-8.

28. Schuchardt JP, Schneider I, Meyer H, et al. Incorporation of EPA and DHA into plasma phospholipids in response to different omega-3 fatty acid formulations--a comparative bioavailability study of fish oil vs. krill oil. *Lipids Health Dis.* 2011 Aug 22;10:145.

29. Neubronner J, Schuchardt JP, Kressel G, et al. Enhanced increase of omega-3 index in response to long-term n-3 fatty acid supplementation from triacylglycerides versus ethyl esters. *Eur J Clin Nutr.* 2011 Deb;65(2):247-54.

30. Dyerberg J, Madsen P, Moller JM, et al. Bioavailability of marine n-3 fatty acid formulations. *Prostaglandins Leukot Essent Fatty Acids.* 2010 Sep;83(3):137-41.

31. Krill [Internet]. *Nat Geog.* Available from http://www.nationalgeographic.com /animals/invertebrates/group/krill/.

32. Ulven SM, Kirkhus B, Lamglait A, et al. Metabolic effects of krill oil are essentially similar to those of fish oil but at lower dose of EPA and DHA, in healthy volunteers. *Lipids.* 2011 Jan;46(1):37-46.

33. Nguyen LN, Ma D, Shui G, et al. Mfsd2a is a transporter for the essential omega-3 fatty acid docosahexaenoic acid. *Nature.* 2014 May 22;509(7501):503-6.

34. Alakbarzade V, Hameed A, Quek DQ, et al. A partially inactivating mutation in the sodium-dependent lysophosphatidylcholine transporter MFSD2A causes a non-lethal microcephaly syndrome. *Nat Genet.* 2015 Jul;47(7):814-7.

35. Guemez-Gamboa A, Nguyen LN, Yang H, et al. Inactivating mutations in MFSD2A, required for omega-3 fatty acid transport in brain, cause a lethal microcephaly syndrome. *Nat Genet.* 2015 Jul;47(7):809-13.

36. Nishida Y, Yamashita E, Miki W, et al. Quenching activities of common hydrophilic and lipophilic antioxidants against singlet oxygen using chemiluminescence detection system. *Carotenoid Science.* 2007 Jan;11(6):16-20.

37. Corbin KD, Zeisel SH. Choline metabolism provides novel insights into nonalcoholic fatty liver disease and its progression. *Curr Opin Gastroenterol.* 2012 Mar;28(2):159-65.

38. Nguyen LN, Ma D, Shui G, et al. Mfsd2a is a transporter for the essential omega-3 fatty acid docosahexaenoic acid. *Nature.* 2014 May 22;509(7501):503-6.

39. Alakbarzade V, Hameed A, Quek DQ, et al. A partially inactivating mutation in the sodium-dependent lysophosphatidylcholine transporter MFSD2A causes a non-lethal microcephaly syndrome. *Nat Genet.* 2015 Jul;47(7):814-7.

40. Guemez-Gamboa A, Nguyen LN, Yang H, et al. Inactivating mutations in MFSD2A, required for omega-3 fatty acid transport in brain, cause a lethal microcephaly syndrome. *Nat Genet.* 2015 Jul;47(7):809-13.

41. MSC labelled Aker Biomarine krill products are from a sustainable and well-managed fishery [Internet. *Marine Stewardship Counci.* 2018 Mar 27. Available from http://www.msc.org/newsroom/news/msc-labelled-aker-biomarine-krill -products-are-from-a-sustainable-and-well-managed-fishery.

42. Ulven SM, Kirkhus B, Lamglait A, et al. Metabolic effects of krill oil are essentially similar to those of fish oil but at lower dose of EPA and DHA, in healthy volunteers. *Lipids.* 2011 Jan;46(1):37-46.

43. Krill oil. Monograph. *Altern Med Rev.* 2010 Apr;15(1):84-6.

44. Maki KC, Reeves MS, Farmer M, et al. Krill oil supplementation increases plasma concentrations of eicosapentaenoic and docosahexaenoic acids in overweight and obese men and women. *Nutr Res.* 2009 Sep;29(9):609-15.

45. Deutsch L. Evaluation of the effect of Neptune Krill Oil on chronic inflammation and arthritic symptoms. *J Am Coll Nutr.* 2007 Feb;26(1):39-48.

46. Sampalis F, Bunea R, Pelland MF, et al. Evaluation of the effects of Neptune Krill Oil on the management of premenstrual syndrome and dysmenorrhea. *Altern Med Rev.* 2003 May;8(2):171-9.

47. Gamma-linolenic acid (GLA). Monograph. *Altern Med Rev.* 2004 Mar;9(1):70-8.

48. Ibid.

49. Leventhal LJ, Boyce EG, Zurier RB. Treatment of rheumatoid arthritis with gammalinolenic acid. *Ann Intern Med.* 1993 Nov 1;119(9):867-73.

50. Zurier RB, Rossetti RG, Jacobson EW, et al. gamma-Linolenic acid treatment of rheumatoid arthritis. A randomized, placebo-controlled trial. *Arthritis Rheum.* 1996 Nov;39(11):1808-17.

51. Gamma-linolenic acid (GLA). Monograph. *Altern Med Rev.* 2004 Mar;9(1):70-8.

52. Leventhal LJ, Boyce EG, Zurier RB. Treatment of rheumatoid arthritis with blackcurrant seed oil. *Br J Rheumatol.* 1994 Sep;33(9):847-52.

53. Melnik BC, Plewig G. Is the origin of atopy linked to deficient conversion of omega-6-fatty acids to prostaglandin E1? *J Am Acad Dermatol.* 1989 Sep;21(3 Pt 1):557-63.

54. Morse PF, Horrobin DF, Manku MS, et al. Meta-analysis of placebo-controlled studies of the efficacy of Epogam in the treatment of atopic eczema. Relationship between plasma essential fatty acid changes and clinical response. *Br J Dermatol.* 1989 Jul;121(1):75-90.

55. Horrobin DF. Nutritional and medical importance of gamma-linolenic acid. *Prog Lipid Res.* 1992;31(2):163-94.

56. Hansen AE. Essential fatty acids and infant nutrition; Borden award address. *Pediatrics* 1958 Mar;21(3):494-501.

57. Surette ME, Stull D, Lindemann J. The impact of a medical food containing gammalinolenic and eicosapentaenoic acids on asthma management and the quality of life of adult asthma patients. *Curr Med Res Opin.* 2008 Feb;24(2):559-67.

58. Brush MG, Watson SJ, Horrobin DF, et al. Abnormal essential fatty acid levels in plasma of women with premenstrual syndrome. *Am J Obstet Gynecol.* 1984 Oct;150(4):363-6.

59. Arnold LE, Pinkham SM, Votolato N. Does zinc moderate essential fatty acid and amphetamine treatment of attention-deficit/hyperactivity disorder? *J Child Adolesc Psychopharmacol.* 2000 Summer;10(2):111-7.

60. Kruger MC, Coetzer H, de Winter R, et al. Calcium, gamma-linolenic acid and eicosapentaenoic acid supplementation in senile osteoporosis. *Aging (Milano)*. 1998 Oct;10(5):385-94.

61. Barabino S, Rolando M, Camicione P, et al. Systemic linoleic and gamma-linolenic acid therapy in dry eye syndrome with an inflammatory component. *Cornea*. 2003 Mar;22(2):97-101.

62. Guillaume D, Charrouf Z. Argan oil. Monograph. *Altern Med Rev.* 2011 Sep;16(3):275-9.

63. Charrouf Z, Guillaume D. Should the amazigh diet (regular and moderate argan-oil consumption) have a beneficial impact on human health? *Crit Rev Food Sci Nutr.* 2010 May;50(5):473-7.

64. Guillaume D, Charrouf Z. Argan oil. Monograph. *Altern Med Rev.* 2011 Sep;16(3):275-9.

65. Ibid.

66. Harhar H, Gharby S, Kartah B, et al. Influence of argan kernel roasting-time on virgin argan oil composition and oxidative stability. *Plant Foods Hum Nutr.* 2011 Jan;66(2):163-8.

67. Guillaume D, Charrouf Z. Argan oil. Monograph. *Altern Med Rev.* 2011 Sep;16(3):275-9.

68. Ibid.

69. Dobrev H. Clinical and instrumental study of the efficacy of a new sebum control cream. *J Cosmet Dermatol.* 2007 Jun;6(2):113-8.

70. Berrougui H, Ettaib A, Herrera Gonzalez MD, et al. Hypolipidemic and hypocholesterolemic effect of argan oil (Argania spinosa L.) in Meriones shawi rats. *J Ethnopharmacol.* 2003 Nov;89(1):15-8.

71. Derouiche A, Cherki M, Drissi A, et al. Nutritional intervention study with argan oil in man: effects on lipids and apolipoproteins. *Ann Nutr Metab.* 2005 May-Jun;49(3):196-201.

72. Berrougui H, Cloutier M, Isabelle M, et al. Phenolic-extract from argan oil (Argania spinosa L.) inhibits human low-density lipoprotein (LDL) oxidation and enhances cholesterol efflux from human THP-1 macrophages. *Atherosclerosis.* 2006 Feb;184(2):389-96.

73. Cherki M, Derouiche A, Drissi A, et al. Consumption of argan oil may have an antiatherogenic effect by improving paraoxonase activities and antioxidant status: Intervention study in healthy men. *Nutr Metab Cardiovasc Dis.* 2005 Oct;15(5):352-60.

74. Ould Mohamedou MM, Zouirech K, El Messal M, et al. Argan oil exerts an antiatherogenic effect by improving lipids and susceptibility of LDL to oxidation in type 2 diabetes patients. *Int J Endocrinol.* 2011;2011:747835.

75. Ibid.

76. Haimeur A, Messaouri H, Ulmann L, et al. Argan oil prevents prothrombotic complications by lowering lipid levels and platelet aggregation, enhancing oxidative status in dyslipidemic patients from the area of Rabat (Morocco). *Lipids Health Dis.* 2013;12:107.

77. Ibid.

78. Mekhfi H, Belmekki F, Ziyyat A, et al. Antithrombotic activity of argan oil: an in vivo experimental study. *Nutrition.* 2012 Sep;28(9):937-41.

79. El Midaoui A, Haddad Y, Couture R. Beneficial effects of argan oil on blood pressure, insulin resistance, and oxidative stress in rat. *Nutrition.* 2016 Oct;32(10):1132-7.

80. Bellahcen S, Hakkou Z, Ziyyat A, et al. Antidiabetic and antihypertensive effect of Virgin Argan Oil in model of neonatal streptozotocin-induced diabetic and l-nitroarginine methylester (l-NAME) hypertensive rats. *J Complement Integr Med.* 2013 Jul 6;10.

81. Berrougui H, Alvarez de Sotomayor M, Perez-Guerrero C, et al. Argan (Argania spinosa) oil lowers blood pressure and improves endothelial dysfunction in spontaneously hypertensive rats. *Br J Nutr.* 2004 Dec;92(6):921-9.

82. Berrada Y, Settaf A, Baddouri K, et al. [Experimental evidence of an antihypertensive and hypocholesterolemic effect of oil of argan, Argania sideroxylon]. *Therapie.* 2000 May-Jun;55(3):375-8.

83. Guillaume D, Charrouf Z. Argan oil. Monograph. *Altern Med Rev.* 2011 Sep;16(3):275-9.

Chapter 9

1. Daley CA, Abbott A, Doyle PS, et al. A review of fatty acid profiles and antioxidant content in grass-fed and grain-fed beef. *Nutr J.* 2010 Mar;9:10.

2. Moyad MA. An introduction to dietary/supplemental omega-3 fatty acids for general health and prevention: part I. *Urol Oncol.* 2005 Jan-Feb;23(1):28-35.

3. Arab-Tehrany E, Jacquot M, Gaiani C, et al. Beneficial effects and oxidative stability of omega-3 long-chain polyunsaturated fatty acids. *Trends in Food Science & Technology.* 2012 May;25(1):24-33.

4. Modified from Arab-Tehrany E, Jacquot M, Gaiani C, et al. Beneficial effects and oxidative stability of omega-3 long-chain polyunsaturated fatty acids. *Trends in Food Science & Technology.* 2012 May;25(1):24-33.

5. How safe is your shrimp? [Internet]. *Consumer Reports.* 2015 Apr 24 [cited 4 Jun 2018]. Available from http://www.consumerreports.org/cro/magazine/2015/06/shrimp-safety/index.htm.

6. Wild caught vs. farm raised [Internet]. *Carson & Co.* [cited 4 Jun 2018]. Available from http://www.carsonandcompany.net/shrimp-products/wild-caught-shrimp-vs-farm-raised.

7. Au WW. Susceptibility of children to environmental toxic substances. *Int J Hyg Env Health.* 2002; 205(1). Available from http://www.citizen.org/cmep/article_redirect.cfm?ID=12706.

8. DiNicolantonio JJ, McCarty MF, Chatterjee S, et al. A higher dietary ratio of long-chain omega-3 to total omega-6 fatty acids for prevention of COX-2-dependent adenocarcinomas. *Nutr Cancer.* 2014;66(8):1279-84.

9. *Selfnutritiondata.* http://nutritiondata.self.com. Accessed 2/12/2018.

10. Herrera-Camacho J, Soberano-Martinez A, Orozco Duran KE. Effect of fatty acids on reproductive performance of ruminants. *Artificial Insemination in Farm Animals.* 2011 Jun 21:217-242. Available at http://www.intechopen.com /books/artificial-insemination-in-farm-animals/effect-of-fatty-acids-on -reproductive-performance-of-ruminants.

11. *USDA Food Composition Databases* [Internet]. Available from https://ndb.nal .usda.gov/ndb/.

12. Adapted from Rodriguez-Leyva D, Dupasquier CM, McCullough R, et al. The cardiovascular effects of flaxseed and its omega-3 fatty acid, alpha-linolenic acid. *Can J Cardiol.* 2010 Nov;26(9):489-96.

13. James MJ, Gibson RA, Cleland LG. Dietary polyunsaturated fatty acids and inflammatory mediator production. *Am J Clin Nutr.* 2000 Jan;71(1 Suppl):343s-8s.

14. Rallidis LS, Paschos G, Liakos GK, et al. Dietary alpha-linolenic acid decreases C-reactive protein, serum amyloid A and interleukin-6 in dyslipidaemic patients. *Atherosclerosis.* 2003 Apr;167(2):237-42.

15. Paschos GK, Rallidis LS, Liakos GK, et al. Background diet influences the anti-inflammatory effect of alpha-linolenic acid in dyslipidaemic subjects. *Br J Nutr.* 2004 Oct;92(4):649-55.

16. Bemelmans WJ, Lefrandt JD, Feskens EJ, et al. Increased alpha-linolenic acid intake lowers C-reactive protein, but has no effect on markers of atherosclerosis. *Eur J Clin Nutr.* 2004 Jul;58(7):1083-9.

17. Allman MA, Pena MM, Pang D. Supplementation with flaxseed oil versus sunflowerseed oil in healthy young men consuming a low fat diet: effects on platelet composition and function. *Eur J Clin Nutr.* 1995 Mar;49(3):169-78.

18. Zhao G, Etherton TD, Martin KR, et al. Dietary alpha-linolenic acid reduces inflammatory and lipid cardiovascular risk factors in hypercholesterolemic men and women. *J Nutr.* 2004 Nov;134(11):2991-7.

19. Faintuch J, Horie LM, Barbeiro HV, et al. Systemic inflammation in morbidly obese subjects: response to oral supplementation with alpha-linolenic acid. *Obes Surg.* 2007 Mar;17(3):341-7.

20. Mandasescu S, Mocanu V, Dascalita AM, et al. Flaxseed supplementation in hyperlipidemic patients. *Rev Med Chir Soc Med Nat Iasi.* 2005 Jul-Sep;109(3):502-6.

21. Bloedon LT, Balikai S, Chittams J, et al. Flaxseed and cardiovascular risk factors: results from a double blind, randomized, controlled clinical trial. *J Am Coll Nutr.* 2008 Feb;27(1):65-74.

22. Mandasescu S, Mocanu V, Dascalita AM, et al. Flaxseed supplementation in hyperlipidemic patients. *Rev Med Chir Soc Med Nat Iasi.* 2005 Jul-Sep;109(3):502-6.

23. Kawakami Y, Yamanaka-Okumura H, Naniwa-Kuroki Y, et al. Flaxseed oil intake reduces serum small dense low-density lipoprotein concentrations in Japanese men: a randomized, double blind, crossover study. *Nutr J.* 2015 Apr 21;14:39.

24. Bassett CM, McCullough RS, Edel AL, et al. The alpha-linolenic acid content of flaxseed can prevent the atherogenic effects of dietary trans fat. *Am J Physiol Heart Circ Physiol* 2011;301:H2220-6.

25. Manda D, Giurcaneanu G, Ionescu L, et al. Lipid profile after alpha-linolenic acid (ALA) enriched eggs diet: a study on healthy volunteers. *Archiva Zootechnica.* 2008;11(2):35-41.

26. Daley CA, Abbott A, Doyle PS, et al. A review of fatty acid profiles and antioxidant content in grass-fed and grain-fed beef. *Nutr J.* 2010 Mar;9:10.

27. Ibid.

28. Pariza MW, Park Y, Cook ME. Mechanisms of action of conjugated linoleic acid: evidence and speculation. *Proc Soc Exp Biol Med.* 2000 Jan;223(1):8-13.

29. Moon HS. Biological effects of conjugated linoleic acid on obesity-related cancers. *Chem Biol Interact.* 2014 Dec 5;224:189-95.

30. Daley CA, Abbott A, Doyle PS, et al. A review of fatty acid profiles and antioxidant content in grass-fed and grain-fed beef. *Nutrition Journal.* 2010;9:10.

31. Dhiman TR, Anand GR, Satter LD, et al. Conjugated linoleic acid content of milk from cows fed different diets. *J Dairy Sci.* 1999 Oct;82(1):2146-56.

32. Lehnen TE, da Silva MR, Camacho A, et al. A review on effects of conjugated linoleic fatty acid (CLA) upon body composition and energetic metabolism. *J Int Soc Sports Nutr.* 2015;12:36.

33. McCrorie TA, Keaveney EM, Wallace JM, et al. Human health effects of conjugated linoleic acid from milk and supplements. *Nutr Res Rev.* 2011 Dec;24(2):206-27.

34. Gaullier JM, Halse J, Hoivik HO, et al. Six months supplementation with conjugated linoleic acid induces regional-specific fat mass decreases in overweight and obese. *Br J Nutr.* 2007 Mar;97(3):550-60.

35. Wang Y, Jones PJ. Dietary conjugated linoleic acid and body composition. *Am J Clin Nutr.* 2004 Jun;79(6 Suppl):1153s-8s.

36. Daley CA, Abbott A, Doyle PS, et al. A review of fatty acid profiles and antioxidant content in grass-fed and grain-fed beef. *Nutr J.* 2010 Mar;9:10.

37. Ibid.

38. Ibid.

39. Ibid.

40. Descalzo AM, Rossetti L, Grigioni G, et al. Antioxidant status and odour profile in fresh beef from pasture or grain-fed cattle. *Meat Sci.* 2007 Feb;75(2):299-307.

41. Gatellier P, Mercier Y, Renerre M. Effect of diet finishing mode (pasture or mixed diet) on antioxidant status of Charolais bovine meat. *Meat Sci.* 2004 Jul;67(3):385-94.

42. Daley CA, Abbott A, Doyle PS, et al. A review of fatty acid profiles and antioxidant content in grass-fed and grain-fed beef. *Nutr J.* 2010 Mar;9:10.

43. Mercola J. The unsavory aspects of farmed shrimp [Internet]. *Mercola*. 2013 Aug 14 [cited 4 Jun 2018]. Available from http://articles.mercola.com/sites/articles/archive/2013/08/14/farmed-shrimp.aspx.

44. How safe is your shrimp? [Internet]. *Consumer Reports*. 2015 Apr 24 [cited 4 Jun 2018]. Available from http://www.consumerreports.org/cro/magazine/2015/06/shrimp-safety/index.htm.

45. Gunnars K. Grass-fed vs. grain-fed beef—what's the difference? [Internet]. *Healthline*. 2018 May 7 [cited 4 Jun 2018]. Available from https://authoritynutrition.com/grass-fed-vs-grain-fed-beef/.

46. Robinson J. Health benefits of grass-fed products [Internet]. *Eatwild*. [cited 4 Jun 2018]. Available from http://www.eatwild.com/healthbenefits.htm.

47. Ibid.

48. Chicken, broilers or fryers, back, meat and skin, cooked, rotisserie, original seasoning [Internet]. *Selfnutritiondata* [cited 4 Jun 2018]. Available from. http://nutritiondata.self.com/facts/poultry-products/10483/2.

49. Pork, fresh, loin, blade (chops), bone-in, separable lean and fat, cooked, braised [Internet]. *Selfnutritiondata* [cited 4 Jun 2018]. Available from http://nutritiondata.self.com/facts/pork-products/2120/2.

50. Beef, tenderloin, separable lean and fat, trimmed to 0" fat, all grades, cooked, broiled [Internet]. *Selfnutritiondata* [cited 4 Jun 2018]. Available from http://nutritiondata.self.com/facts/beef-products/3574/2.

INDEX

NOTE: Page references in *italics* refer to figures.

C

D

ACKNOWLEDGMENTS

Nils Hoem and Jake Toughill—your contributions to this book were invaluable.

— Dr. DiNicolantonio

Dr. Nils Hoem, the chief scientist for Aker Biomarine, for all his technical assistance on omega-3.

— Dr. Mercola

ABOUT THE AUTHORS

Dr. Joseph Mercola is a physician and *New York Times* best-selling author. He was voted the Ultimate Wellness Game Changer by the Huffington Post and has been featured in several national media outlets, including *Time* magazine, the *Los Angeles Times*, CNN, Fox News, ABC News, *TODAY*, and *The Dr. Oz Show*. His mission is to transform the traditional medical paradigm in the United States into one in which the root cause of disease is treated, rather than the symptoms. In addition, he aims to expose corporate and government fraud and mass media hype that often sends people down an unhealthy path.

James J. DiNicolantonio, Pharm.D., is a cardiovascular research scientist and doctor of pharmacy at Saint Luke's Mid America Heart Institute in Kansas City, Missouri. A well-respected and internationally known scientist and expert on health and nutrition, he has contributed extensively to health policy and has testified in front of the Canadian Senate regarding the harms of added sugars. He is the author of *The Salt Fix*. Dr. DiNicolantonio serves as the Associate Editor of *Nutrition* and British Medical Journal's (BMJ) *Open Heart*, a journal published in partnership with the British Cardiovascular Society. He is the author or coauthor of approximately 200 publications in the medical literature. He is also on the editorial advisory boards of several other medical journals.

Hay House Titles of Related Interest

YOU CAN HEAL YOUR LIFE, the movie, starring Louise Hay & Friends
(available as a 1-DVD program, an expanded 2-DVD set, and an online
streaming video)
Learn more at www.hayhouse.com/louise-movie

THE SHIFT, the movie,
starring Dr. Wayne W. Dyer
(available as a 1-DVD program, an expanded 2-DVD set, and an online
streaming video)
Learn more at www.hayhouse.com/the-shift-movie

⁓

*THE ALLERGY SOLUTION: Unlock the Surprising Hidden Truth about
Why You Are Sick and How to Get Well,* by Leo Galland, M.D.,
and Jonathan Galland, J.D.

*CULTURED FOOD IN A JAR: 100+ Probiotic Recipes to Inspire
and Change Your Life,* by Donna Schwenk

*THE DENTAL DIET: The Surprising Link between Your Teeth, Real Food,
and Life-Changing Natural Health,* by Dr. Steven Lin

*OUTSIDE THE BOX CANCER THERAPIES: Alternative Therapies That Treat
and Prevent Cancer,* by Dr. Mark Stengler and Dr. Paul Anderson

*THE REAL FOOD REVOLUTION: Healthy Eating, Green Groceries, and the
Return of the American Family Farm,* by Congressman Tim Ryan

All of the above are available at your local bookstore,
or may be ordered by contacting Hay House (see next page).

⁓

We hope you enjoyed this Hay House book. If you'd like to receive our online catalog featuring additional information on Hay House books and products, or if you'd like to find out more about the Hay Foundation, please contact:

Hay House, Inc., P.O. Box 5100, Carlsbad, CA 92018-5100
(760) 431-7695 or (800) 654-5126
(760) 431-6948 (fax) or (800) 650-5115 (fax)
www.hayhouse.com® • www.hayfoundation.org

———

Published in Australia by:
Hay House Australia Pty. Ltd., 18/36 Ralph St., Alexandria NSW 2015
Phone: 612-9669-4299 • *Fax:* 612-9669-4144 • www.hayhouse.com.au

Published in the United Kingdom by:
Hay House UK, Ltd., Astley House, 33 Notting Hill Gate, London W11 3JQ
Phone: 44-20-3675-2450 • *Fax:* 44-20-3675-2451 • www.hayhouse.co.uk

Published in India by: Hay House Publishers India,
Muskaan Complex, Plot No. 3, B-2, Vasant Kunj, New Delhi 110 070
Phone: 91-11-4176-1620 • *Fax:* 91-11-4176-1630 • www.hayhouse.co.in

———

Access New Knowledge.
Anytime. Anywhere.

Learn and evolve at your own pace
with the world's leading experts.

www.hayhouseU.com